I0705351

Introduction

In the modern workplace, success is often measured by productivity, efficiency, and output. We sit for hours on end, glued to our screens, racing against deadlines, and often pushing ourselves to the limit—all in pursuit of career growth and achievement. However, in this relentless drive for progress, we often overlook a crucial element that directly impacts not only our performance but also our long-term well-being: **our physical health**.

The workplace has evolved dramatically over the past few decades, with technological advancements allowing us to work faster and smarter. But with these changes has come an unintended consequence—**a sedentary office culture**. From long hours at our desks to virtual meetings that demand little more than a few clicks, many of us are spending the majority of our day sitting, leading to a lifestyle that lacks the movement our bodies desperately need.

The shift toward a more sedentary work environment might seem harmless at first glance, but it's a problem that has significant health implications. Sitting for extended periods has been linked to a host of serious conditions, including heart disease, diabetes, obesity, and even certain types of cancer. What's more, a lack of movement can impact mental health, contributing to increased stress, anxiety, and decreased productivity. For all the benefits that come with modern work environments, the cost of neglecting our physical well-being can be incredibly high.

This book, **Workplace Wellness: Thriving Through Fitness at the Office**, is designed to be your guide to **breaking free from the sedentary trap** and reclaiming your health without sacrificing your professional success. It's about rethinking how we work, not just for greater productivity, but for improved physical and mental well-being.

In these pages, you'll discover practical strategies to incorporate movement into your workday, reduce the harmful effects of prolonged sitting, and improve your overall fitness. Whether you work in a traditional office, from home, or in a hybrid environment, this book will show you how to create a healthier routine that fits seamlessly into your work life. You don't need to overhaul your day or spend hours in the gym—small changes can have a profound impact.

We'll explore everything from **desk exercises and ergonomic setups** to **managing stress through fitness** and building a culture of wellness in the workplace. Along the way, you'll gain insight into the science behind movement, understand the risks of a sedentary lifestyle, and learn how to overcome common barriers to staying active in the office.

No matter your role, schedule, or current fitness level, **Workplace Wellness** is here to help you unlock the potential of an active, healthy, and fulfilling work life. The journey toward a more energized, productive, and healthier you begins with the small steps outlined in this book—steps that can easily be integrated into even the busiest of workdays.

It's time to stop seeing fitness and work as separate parts of your life and start embracing the idea that movement is a key component to both your professional success and personal health. With the tools and knowledge in this book, you'll be ready to transform your workplace habits and take control of your well-being—without sacrificing your productivity or your goals.

Welcome to a healthier way to work. Let's get started.

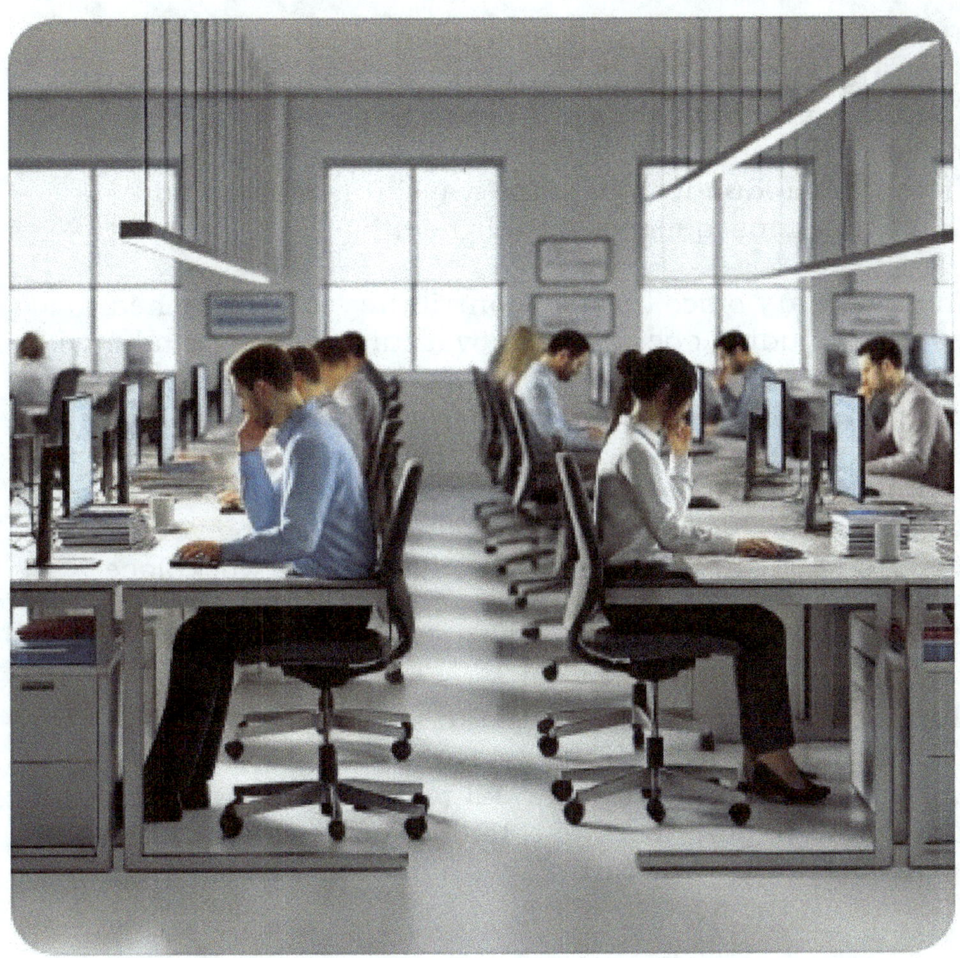

Chapter 1: The Sedentary Office Lifestyle

The Modern Office: A Sedentary Trap

In recent decades, the way we work has undergone a dramatic transformation. Earlier generations often engaged in jobs that required some level of physical activity, such as farming, manufacturing, or walking between workspaces. However, the rise of technology and automation has led to a sharp increase in desk-based jobs, where most workers spend the majority of their day seated. This shift from physical movement to sedentary desk work has created what we now call the "sedentary office lifestyle."

It's easy to fall into this trap of prolonged sitting without realizing the harmful effects. From sitting at the computer, attending meetings, or even commuting, we often find ourselves immobile for hours. While this lifestyle has increased productivity in some ways, it has also had significant consequences on our health.

The sedentary office lifestyle contributes to various health issues, including obesity, cardiovascular disease, and a wide range of musculoskeletal problems. In this chapter, we will explore the science behind the dangers of prolonged sitting and the various ways it can negatively affect both physical and mental well-being. We will also look at simple strategies to combat the harmful effects of sitting, allowing you to maintain your health and productivity in the workplace.

The Science Behind Sitting: How It Affects the Body

Human beings are not designed to sit for long periods. Our ancestors spent most of their day moving—hunting, gathering, or performing manual tasks that required regular movement. In stark contrast, today's office worker may spend up to 10 hours sitting, with limited physical activity throughout the day.

Prolonged sitting affects the body in numerous ways:

1. **Metabolism Slows Down**: When we sit, our calorie burn rate drops significantly, which can lead to weight gain. Sitting also reduces the body's ability to regulate blood sugar and metabolize fat, increasing the risk of metabolic disorders.
2. **Circulation Decreases**: Prolonged sitting causes blood circulation to slow down, particularly in the legs. This can lead to swollen ankles, poor circulation, and an increased risk of blood clots.
3. **Muscles Weaken**: Sitting for long periods leads to muscle inactivity. Muscles such as the glutes, hamstrings, and core become weak, while the hip flexors tighten. This imbalance in muscle use can

contribute to posture problems, back pain, and overall weakness.

4. **Posture Suffers**: Most people don't sit with perfect posture for long periods. Over time, the slouching and forward-leaning that often accompany sitting can lead to spinal misalignment and chronic pain, particularly in the lower back and neck.

The Hidden Dangers of Sitting: A Closer Look at Health Risks

1. Cardiovascular Disease and Metabolic Syndrome

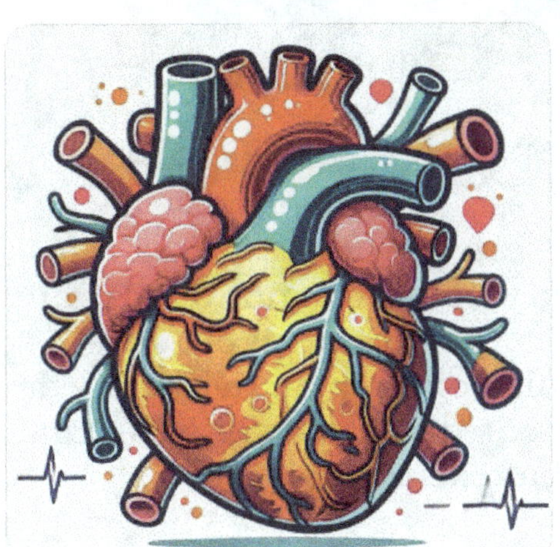

One of the most serious risks of a sedentary lifestyle is the increased risk of cardiovascular disease. Sitting for long hours each day slows down metabolism and decreases insulin sensitivity, leading to higher levels of blood sugar and cholesterol. These changes can contribute to conditions like high blood pressure, heart disease, and even stroke.

Metabolic syndrome—a group of conditions that includes high blood pressure, high blood sugar, and unhealthy cholesterol levels—is also closely linked to prolonged sitting. Individuals with metabolic syndrome are at a significantly higher risk of heart disease, type 2 diabetes, and other serious health conditions.

2. Obesity and Weight Gain

When we sit for long periods, our bodies burn fewer calories than when we're standing or moving. This reduction in calorie expenditure can lead to gradual weight gain, even for individuals who eat relatively healthy diets. Moreover, long periods of inactivity can lead to fat accumulation, particularly around the abdomen, which is a major risk factor for various chronic diseases.

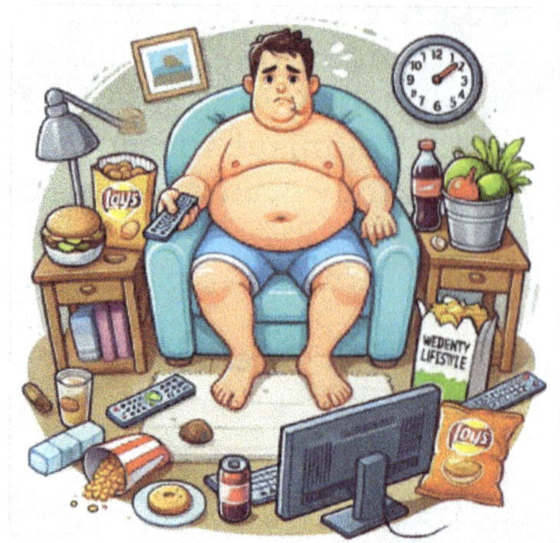

The connection between sedentary behavior and weight gain is strong, and it contributes to the global rise in obesity rates. Even if you engage in regular physical activity outside of work, sitting for extended periods during the day can undo much of the positive effects of that exercise.

3. Musculoskeletal Problems: Back, Neck, and Shoulder Pain

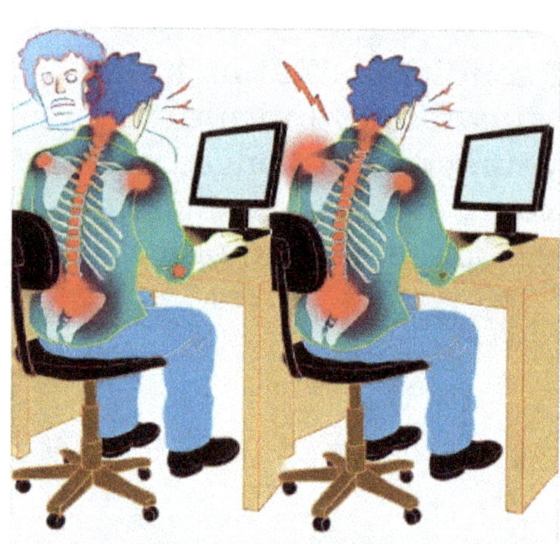

Prolonged sitting puts immense strain on the musculoskeletal system, particularly the back, neck, and shoulders. These areas are prone to pain and injury due to poor posture, lack of movement, and repetitive tasks performed at a desk.

The Spine and Lower Back

When you sit for long periods, particularly with poor posture, you place excessive pressure on the lumbar spine (lower back). This can compress the discs between the vertebrae, leading to **disc degeneration**, bulging, or even herniation. Sitting also weakens the core muscles that support the spine, contributing to lower back pain and increased risk of injury.

The Neck

Forward head posture, often caused by looking at a computer screen, can strain the cervical spine (neck). Known as **tech neck**, this posture causes the head to lean forward, placing additional pressure on the neck and upper spine. For every inch the head moves forward, an extra 10 pounds of pressure is placed on the neck. Over time, this can lead to chronic pain, stiffness, and headaches.

The Shoulders and Upper Back

Rounded shoulders are a common issue among office workers. When the shoulders roll forward while sitting, it shortens the chest muscles and weakens the muscles between the shoulder blades. This imbalance can lead to **shoulder impingement**, upper back pain, and stiffness in the trapezius and rhomboid muscles.

4. Increased Risk of Certain Cancers

Prolonged sitting has been linked to an increased risk of certain cancers, including colon, breast, and endometrial cancers. The exact reasons for this connection are still being studied, but one theory suggests that prolonged sitting leads to increased levels of insulin and inflammation, both of which can promote the growth of cancer cells.

The negative effects of a sedentary lifestyle a ren't limited to physical health. Sitting for long periods can also affect cognitive function and mental well-being. Physical activity helps increase blood flow to the brain, which enhances memory, concentration, and mental clarity. When we remain inactive for long periods, cognitive function declines, leading to **brain fog** and decreased productivity.

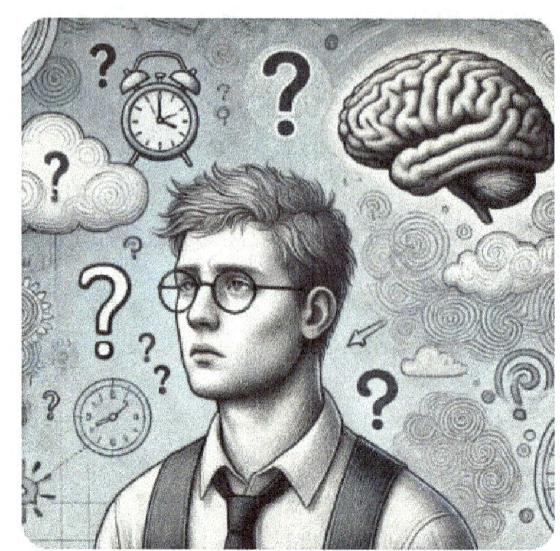

There is also a strong link between sedentary behavior and mental health conditions such as **anxiety** and **depression**. Physical movement releases endorphins—our body's natural mood boosters. When we sit for too long without moving, we miss out on these benefits, potentially leading to increased stress, low energy, and a sense of detachment.

The Impact on Workplace Productivity

Sitting for extended periods doesn't just harm your health—it also affects your productivity. Employees who sit for long periods often report feeling more fatigued, mentally drained, and less engaged with their work. This mental and physical stagnation leads to:

- **Lower Energy Levels**: Prolonged sitting causes fatigue, contributing to the dreaded afternoon slump.
- **Reduced Focus**: When we sit for too long, the brain's supply of oxygen and blood flow decreases, leading to a decline in focus and concentration.
- **Increased Risk of Errors**: Fatigue and poor concentration can lead to more mistakes and a decrease in work quality.

Fortunately, by incorporating movement into the workday, these issues can be significantly reduced, leading to better performance, creativity, and engagement.

Breaking the Sedentary Cycle: How to Add Movement to Your Day

The dangers of prolonged sitting are real, but the good news is that small, consistent changes can make a significant difference in combating the risks. The key is to add movement to your workday in ways that are both practical and sustainable.

1. Stand Up Regularly

Make it a habit to stand up and stretch at least every 30 minutes. Even short breaks can help reduce the harmful effects of sitting. Set a timer on your phone or use a reminder app to keep yourself on track.

2. Try a Standing Desk

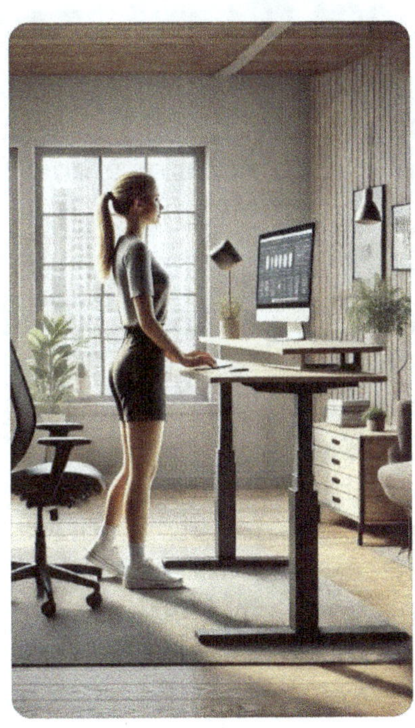

Standing desks are becoming increasingly popular in offices, and for good reason. Alternating between sitting and standing throughout the day can reduce the strain on your spine and muscles, increase calorie burn, and boost energy levels. If a standing desk isn't available, consider using a desk converter that allows you to elevate your monitor and keyboard.

3. Take Walking Breaks

Whenever possible, take a short walk, even if it's just around your office or to grab a coffee. Walking meetings are another great way to add movement to your day while still being productive.

4. Incorporate Desk Stretches

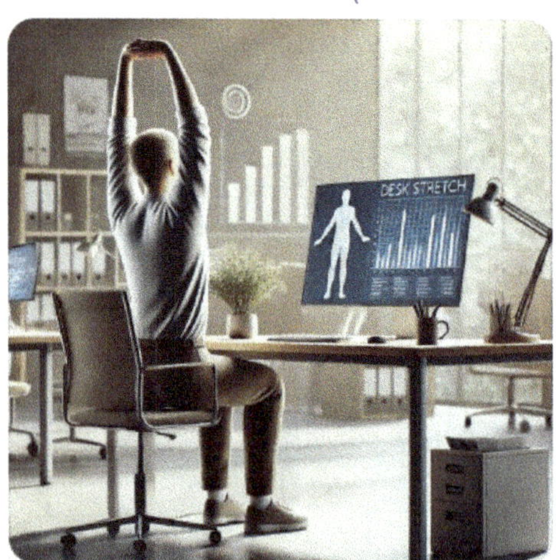

Simple stretches at your desk, such as neck rolls, shoulder shrugs, and seated twists, can help alleviate tension and improve flexibility. These movements can be done in just a few minutes and are a great way to reset your body.

5. Use Active Sitting

If you can't stand or walk during certain tasks, consider active sitting options, such as using a stability ball or a chair that encourages dynamic movement. These tools engage your core and promote better posture, even while seated.

The Importance of Intentional Movement

It's not just about finding time for exercise outside of work—it's about **incorporating intentional movement throughout your workday**. Even if you hit the gym after hours, the harmful effects of sitting can accumulate if you're not moving during the day. The goal is to make movement a natural part of your routine, improving both your physical health and your productivity.

The sedentary office lifestyle is a significant threat to both health and productivity, but it doesn't have to be a permanent part of your workday. By understanding the dangers of prolonged sitting and taking small, manageable steps to incorporate movement, you can break free from the sedentary cycle. In the next chapter, we'll explore more practical ways to combat workplace stress and create an environment that fosters both physical and mental well-being.

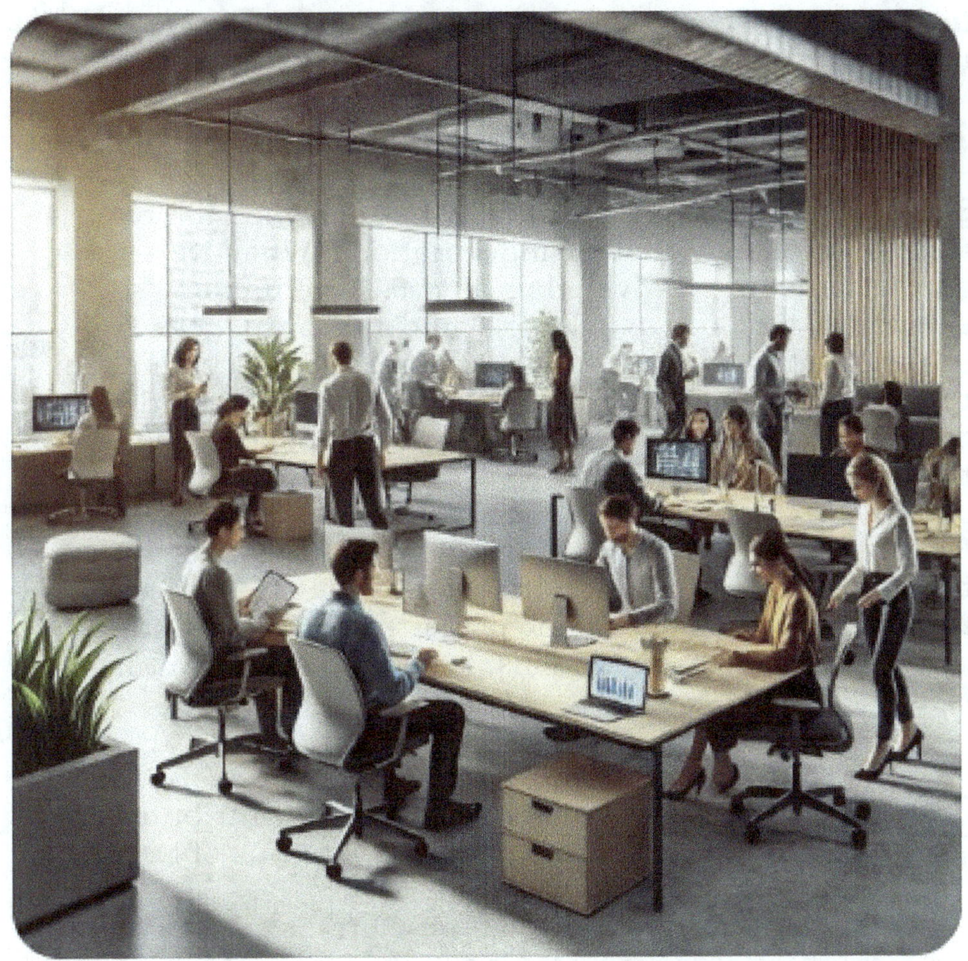

Chapter 2: Understanding Workplace Stress

In the modern workplace, stress has become almost unavoidable. With tight deadlines, high expectations, and increasingly complex workloads, employees face various pressures that can often feel overwhelming. Stress can be a powerful motivator, but chronic, unmanaged stress takes a significant toll on both mental and physical health, affecting productivity, satisfaction, and overall quality of life. In this chapter, we will explore the root causes of workplace stress, its impact on health, and how physical activity and intentional fitness practices can help mitigate stress and improve resilience. By addressing workplace stress holistically, we can foster a healthier, more productive, and more balanced work environment.

The Science of Stress: How It Affects the Body and Mind

Stress is a natural biological response designed to help us react to threats or challenging situations. When we encounter a stressor, whether physical, mental, or emotional, the body's "fight-or-flight" response kicks in, releasing stress hormones like cortisol and adrenaline. This response increases heart rate, sharpens focus, and diverts energy to essential muscles to help us respond to the perceived threat.

However, in a workplace setting, where stressors are often ongoing, this response can lead to chronic stress, keeping the body in a prolonged state of alertness. Chronic stress disrupts various body systems, leading to significant health issues such as:

1. **Cardiovascular Strain**: Prolonged release of stress hormones raises blood pressure and contributes to arterial inflammation, increasing the risk of heart disease and hypertension.
2. **Weakened Immune System**: Chronic stress dampens immune response, making individuals more susceptible to colds, flu, and other infections. Over time, this compromised immunity can lead to more severe health problems.
3. **Digestive Distress**: Stress can disrupt the digestive system, resulting in symptoms like nausea, stomach cramps, bloating, or irritable bowel syndrome (IBS). High stress levels can also lead to overeating or undereating as a coping mechanism.
4. **Mental Health Disorders**: Long-term stress is a significant contributor to anxiety, depression, and burnout. Chronic stress leads to irritability, difficulty focusing, and even feelings of hopelessness, impacting overall quality of life.

Every workplace and job role is unique, but some common sources of stress are universal across industries. Identifying these stressors is essential for creating a personalized plan to reduce stress and maintain a healthy balance between work and personal life. Key sources of workplace stress include:

1. **Workload and Deadlines**: When employees are consistently given more work than they can reasonably complete, it creates a constant state of pressure. Excessive workload without adequate support or resources can lead to chronic stress, resentment, and eventual burnout.
2. **Job Security Concerns**: Fear of layoffs, restructuring, or instability within a company can create anxiety and uncertainty, leading employees to feel insecure about their future and putting additional strain on their mental health.
3. **Poor Work-Life Balance**: With the increased prevalence of remote work and 24/7 connectivity, the line between work and personal life has blurred. Many employees struggle to disconnect from work, leading to a lack of downtime and mental recovery.
4. **Limited Control and Autonomy**: Employees who feel they have little control over their tasks or are micromanaged may experience higher levels of stress. A lack of autonomy can lead to disengagement and a reduced sense of satisfaction in their work.
5. **Interpersonal Conflicts**: Conflicts with coworkers, supervisors, or clients can create a tense work environment and add emotional stress. Frequent misunderstandings or lack of communication can contribute to feelings of isolation and frustration.
6. **Information Overload and Decision Fatigue**: In fast-paced environments, employees are often bombarded with emails, notifications, and a constant influx of information. This can lead to decision fatigue, where

the mental energy required to make decisions depletes over time, increasing stress and reducing efficiency.

The Physical and Mental Impact of Chronic Workplace Stress

Chronic stress is a silent health risk that affects nearly every part of the body, from physical endurance to cognitive abilities. Below are some of the most common physical and mental health impacts of chronic stress:

1. **Burnout and Fatigue**: Chronic stress drains the body's energy reserves, leading to feelings of exhaustion that don't improve with rest. Burnout, often the result of prolonged stress, is characterized by emotional, physical, and mental exhaustion and a decreased sense of accomplishment.
2. **Sleep Disruptions**: High-stress levels can interfere with sleep quality and duration, leading to insomnia, difficulty staying asleep, or non-restorative sleep. Poor sleep not only impairs productivity but also negatively affects mood, memory, and cognitive function.
3. **Cognitive Impairments**: Chronic stress impairs concentration, decision-making, and memory. Stress hormones affect brain function, making it harder to focus on tasks or retain information, leading to a drop in productivity and more frequent errors.
4. **Reduced Social Engagement**: Under chronic stress, individuals may withdraw from social interactions or become irritable and reactive. This impacts workplace relationships, teamwork, and personal relationships outside of work, adding to a sense of isolation.
5. **Increased Physical Health Risks**: Chronic stress can lead to weight gain, high blood pressure, and an increased risk of developing chronic illnesses, such as diabetes and cardiovascular disease, as it encourages unhealthy coping mechanisms like overeating, smoking, or excessive drinking.

One of the most effective ways to manage stress and improve mental well-being is through regular physical activity. Physical activity benefits both the body and mind, helping individuals handle stress more effectively and promoting overall resilience. Here's how fitness acts as a powerful antidote to stress:

1. **Reduces Cortisol and Releases Endorphins**: Exercise reduces cortisol levels, helping the body move away from the "fight-or-flight" response and toward a state of relaxation. It also releases endorphins, which are natural mood lifters that improve outlook and reduce anxiety.
2. **Improves Sleep Quality**: Physical activity can improve both sleep quality and duration, helping individuals feel more rested and resilient. Regular exercise also promotes deep sleep, the most restorative phase of the sleep cycle, essential for stress recovery.
3. **Builds Mental Resilience**: Regular exercise, especially challenging activities like resistance training or high-intensity interval training (HIIT), builds resilience by training both body and mind to overcome obstacles. This strength and endurance translate to handling stress more effectively.
4. **Provides a Healthy Coping Mechanism**: Exercise offers a constructive way to relieve tension and anxiety. Instead of resorting to unhealthy habits like junk food or alcohol, engaging in physical activity provides an outlet for stress that benefits the body and mind.
5. **Boosts Cognitive Function and Focus**: Exercise increases blood flow to the brain, enhancing memory, concentration, and problem-solving skills. This cognitive boost can help individuals feel more in control of tasks, manage stress better, and maintain a positive mindset.

Incorporating fitness into a busy workday doesn't have to mean an intense workout session. Small, intentional activities throughout the day can make a big difference in managing stress. Here are some practical strategies for adding stress-relieving fitness into your daily routine:

1. Mindful Movement Breaks

Incorporate short movement breaks throughout the day to reduce tension and boost energy. Aim to stand, stretch, or take a few steps every 30-60 minutes. Simple desk stretches, such as shoulder rolls, wrist stretches, or standing calf raises, can release tension and keep you engaged.

2. Walking Meetings

Walking meetings are an excellent way to add movement to your day while staying productive. When appropriate, suggest a walking meeting instead of a sit-down one. Walking naturally enhances creativity, encourages open conversation, and reduces the impact of sitting for long periods.

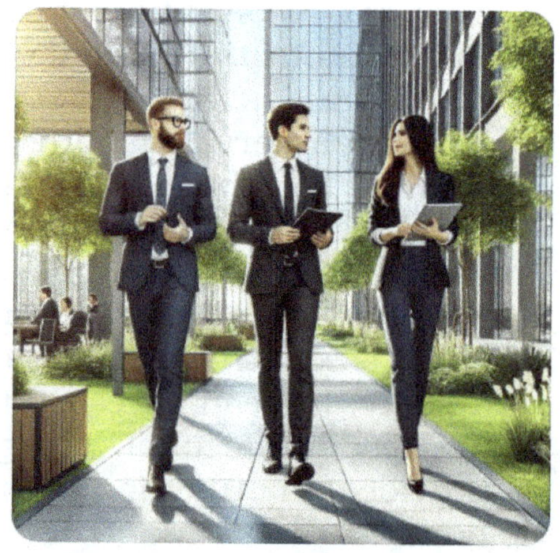

3. Breathing Exercises to Reduce Anxiety

Stress often leads to shallow, rapid breathing, which can exacerbate anxiety. Practicing breathing exercises, such as deep diaphragmatic breathing or box breathing, can help calm the nervous system, reduce anxiety, and increase oxygen flow to the brain. Take a few minutes between tasks to engage in deep breathing for a quick reset.

4. Desk Yoga for Relaxation

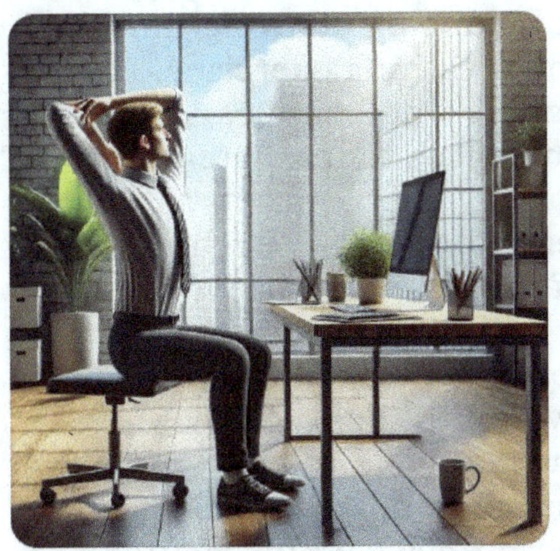

Desk yoga involves simple stretches that can be done at your workstation without taking up much space. Gentle moves like seated twists, neck stretches, and forward folds help relieve tension and promote flexibility. Desk yoga can also improve circulation, refresh the mind, and offer a quick mental break.

5. Lunchtime Physical Activity

If possible, use your lunch break for physical activity. A brisk walk, short workout, or yoga session can break up the day, release pent-up stress, and improve productivity for the afternoon. Even a short walk outside can provide fresh air, sunlight, and a sense of relaxation.

6. Mindfulness and Meditation Practices

Mindfulness exercises, such as meditation, are excellent tools for managing stress. Taking five to ten minutes to focus on your breath, practice mindfulness, or engage in guided meditation can help calm the mind, reduce anxiety, and improve focus. Numerous free apps offer guided meditation, making it easy to incorporate this practice into the workday.

How Employers Can Support Fitness and Stress Management

Employers play a critical role in supporting fitness and wellness in the workplace. When organizations create a culture that prioritizes employee well-being, they foster a healthier, more productive, and more engaged workforce. Here are some ways employers can support stress management and fitness:

1. **Encourage Regular Movement Breaks**: Employers can normalize movement breaks by allowing time for short walks, stretching, or breathing exercises. Creating a culture that values well-being can improve morale and encourage employees to take breaks without guilt.
2. **Provide Access to Fitness Resources**: Organizations can offer on-site fitness facilities, subsidize gym memberships, or provide virtual workout sessions. Making fitness more accessible helps employees incorporate physical activity into their routines.
3. **Organize Wellness Programs**: Wellness programs that include yoga, mindfulness sessions, or fitness challenges can support both physical and mental health. These programs help reduce stress, improve camaraderie, and foster a culture of support.
4. **Promote Work-Life Balance**: Employers can promote work-life balance by offering flexible work schedules, remote work options, or the ability to take longer lunch breaks for exercise. When employees feel supported in balancing work and personal life, they experience reduced stress and greater job satisfaction.

Creating a Personalized Stress Management Plan

Developing a personal plan for managing stress is crucial for long-term well-being. Here are steps to build a personalized strategy:

1. **Identify Stress Triggers**: Knowing the specific causes of your stress allows you to develop targeted coping strategies. Track situations or tasks that trigger stress to understand patterns and find ways to mitigate them.
2. **Incorporate Daily Fitness**: Make movement a non-negotiable part of your day. Even if you can't dedicate

time to a full workout, short movement breaks or stretches can make a big difference in managing stress levels.

3. **Prioritize Self-Care**: Regular self-care activities, such as adequate sleep, healthy eating, and time for relaxation, help build resilience and reduce stress.
4. **Practice Time Management**: Good time management helps reduce last-minute stress and allows you to complete tasks efficiently. Break projects into smaller, manageable parts, prioritize tasks, and avoid overloading your schedule.
5. **Build a Support System**: A strong support network of coworkers, friends, or family provides encouragement and a listening ear. Surround yourself with people who uplift you and offer support, particularly during challenging times.

While workplace stress is common, it doesn't have to dictate your well-being. By understanding the causes and effects of stress, you can take meaningful steps to manage it effectively. Incorporating regular physical activity and building a personal stress management plan are powerful ways to reduce stress, enhance resilience, and maintain a positive mindset in your work life. In the next chapter, we'll explore ergonomics and workspace design, helping you set up an environment that reduces strain, prevents discomfort, and boosts productivity.

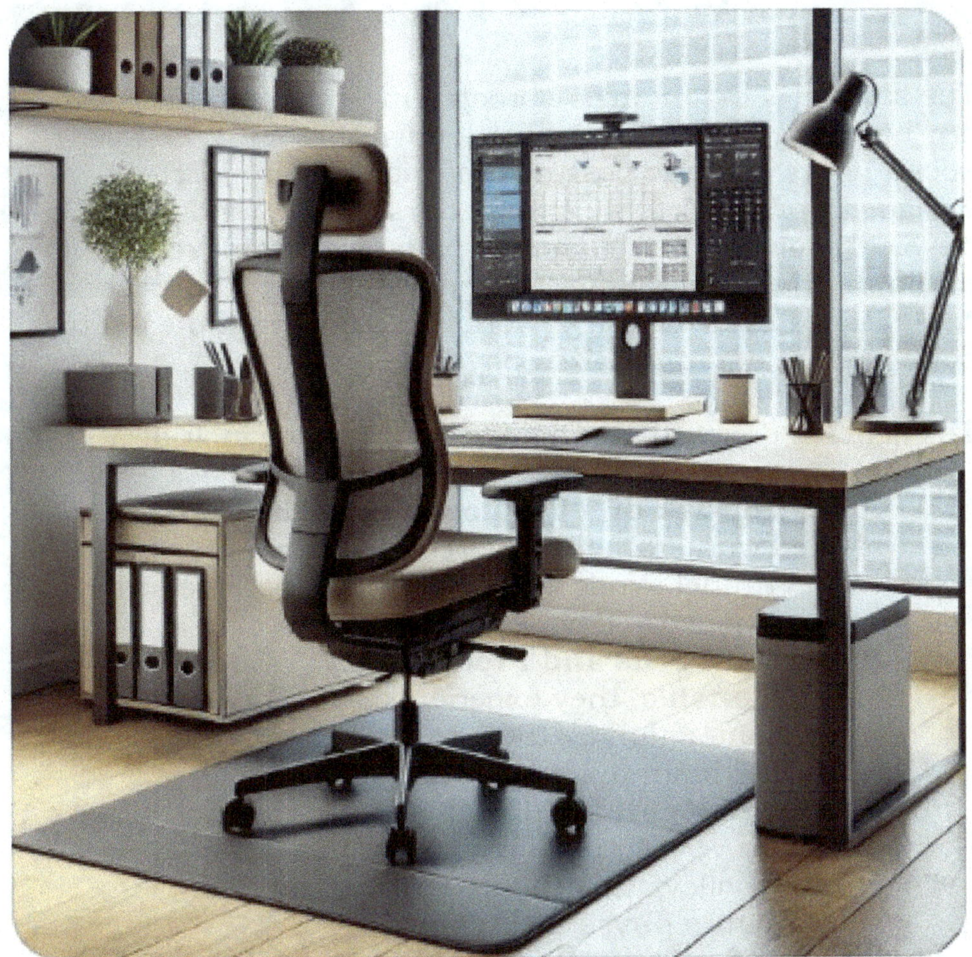

Chapter 3: Ergonomics and Workspace Setup

As the demands of the modern workplace evolve, so does our need for a workspace that prioritizes comfort, efficiency, and well-being. Proper ergonomics—designing a workspace to fit the user—has become essential, especially in office settings where many employees spend long hours sitting in front of screens. An ergonomic workspace not only reduces strain and prevents discomfort but also boosts productivity, focus, and mental well-being. In this chapter, we delve deeply into the principles of ergonomics, practical steps for creating a supportive workspace, and ways to incorporate movement into your day for lasting health benefits.

The science of ergonomics is rooted in understanding how our bodies interact with the work environment. When we spend hours in static postures, particularly in poorly designed workspaces, we expose ourselves to a host of physical problems such as back pain, eye strain, repetitive strain injuries, and mental fatigue. Ergonomics addresses these issues by designing a workspace that promotes natural body posture and minimizes physical strain.

The benefits of a well-ergonomized workspace include:

1. **Reduced Risk of Musculoskeletal Disorders**: A well-aligned workstation helps reduce the risk of back pain, carpal tunnel syndrome, and other repetitive strain injuries.
2. **Increased Focus and Productivity**: When employees are comfortable, they experience less physical distraction, enabling them to focus more intently on tasks and maintain a steady workflow.
3. **Enhanced Mental Well-Being**: An ergonomic setup can improve mental clarity, boost mood, and decrease stress by alleviating the frustration that often accompanies physical discomfort.
4. **Support for Long-Term Health**: Ergonomic adjustments reduce the cumulative strain on the body, making it easier to maintain good health over a long career.

Setting Up Your Ergonomic Workspace: Core Components

A truly ergonomic workspace is tailored to each individual, adjusting elements such as the chair, desk, monitor, keyboard, and lighting to support natural movement and posture. Here's a comprehensive look at each component and how to optimize it for maximum comfort and efficiency.

1. The Chair

The chair is one of the most critical elements in an ergonomic setup, as it supports the body's weight and affects posture. A good ergonomic chair provides ample support for the lower back, allows for adjustability, and encourages natural alignment.

- **Lumbar Support**: Look for a chair with adjustable lumbar support that follows the natural curve of your lower back. Proper lumbar support helps maintain a neutral spine position, reducing strain on the lumbar vertebrae.
- **Seat Height**: Adjust the chair height so that your feet rest flat on the floor, with knees at a 90-degree angle. Proper height helps maintain blood circulation in the legs and prevents strain on the lower back.
- **Seat Depth and Width**: The seat should be deep enough to support your thighs without pressing into the back of your knees. Leave about 2-3 inches between the seat's edge and your knees for comfortable circulation.
- **Backrest Angle and Recline**: Set the backrest angle to a slight recline (100-110 degrees). This recline reduces lumbar pressure and promotes better posture, especially during long periods of sitting.
- **Armrests**: Armrests should be adjustable and positioned so that your shoulders are relaxed and your elbows rest comfortably at a 90-degree angle. Proper arm support helps reduce shoulder and upper back tension.

2. Desk and Work Surface

The desk should support all essential items at a comfortable reach, minimizing the need to stretch, lean, or twist. Here's how to optimize desk ergonomics:

- **Desk Height**: The desk should allow your forearms to rest parallel to the ground when using the keyboard.

For most people, a height between 28 and 30 inches works well, but this may vary based on individual proportions.

- **Clearance Under the Desk**: Ensure there is enough space for your legs to move freely under the desk. Cluttered spaces restrict movement and may lead to awkward postures that contribute to discomfort.
- **Organization and Layout**: Keep frequently used items, like your phone, mouse, and notepad, within easy reach to prevent excessive leaning or stretching. Organize less frequently used items to the side or further back to encourage occasional movement and avoid repetitive strain.

3. Monitor Placement

Proper monitor placement is essential to prevent neck strain, eye fatigue, and upper back discomfort. Positioning your monitor correctly will help maintain a natural head position and minimize the need to look up or down.

- **Height**: The top of the monitor should be at or slightly below eye level, allowing you to view the screen with a slight downward gaze. This helps reduce neck strain and prevents "tech neck."
- **Distance**: Place the monitor about an arm's length (20-30 inches) away from your eyes. This distance minimizes eye strain while allowing you to view the screen without leaning forward.
- **Angle**: Tilt the monitor slightly (10-20 degrees) to reduce glare and create a more comfortable viewing angle. If you use bifocals, a slight downward tilt may help align your line of sight.
- **Dual Monitors**: For dual monitors, align both screens side by side at a similar height and angle. If one monitor is used more frequently, place it directly in front of you to reduce repetitive head rotation.

Improper keyboard and mouse positioning can lead to wrist pain, carpal tunnel syndrome, and other repetitive strain injuries. These tools should be positioned to promote a natural wrist posture and easy access.

- **Keyboard Position**: Position the keyboard close enough so that your elbows are at a 90-degree angle, with your wrists straight. The keyboard should be slightly below elbow level to keep your wrists in a neutral position.
- **Wrist Support**: A padded wrist rest can help keep your wrists aligned with your forearms. Avoid bending the wrists up or down, as this increases strain on the tendons and nerves.
- **Mouse Position**: Place the mouse close to the keyboard to prevent overreaching, and consider using an ergonomic mouse to reduce wrist strain. A trackball or vertical mouse can help minimize wrist movement.
- **Keyboard Tilt**: A slight negative tilt (the keyboard angled slightly downward) is ideal for keeping wrists in a neutral position and reducing strain.

5. Lighting and Screen Brightness

Proper lighting reduces eye strain, minimizes glare, and helps maintain focus. Too much brightness can cause discomfort, while insufficient lighting can lead to squinting and eye fatigue.

- **Natural Light**: Arrange your desk to take advantage of natural light without causing screen glare. Exposure to natural light has been shown to improve mood, energy, and productivity.
- **Task Lighting**: Use adjustable task lighting, like a desk lamp, to illuminate documents or tasks without the need for excessive screen brightness. A well-placed light source can reduce eye strain.

- **Screen Brightness and Contrast**: Adjust the monitor's brightness and contrast to match ambient lighting. The screen should be neither too bright nor too dim, as extreme levels cause eye fatigue.

Common Ergonomic Challenges and Solutions

Even with an ergonomic workspace, some common issues may still arise, especially for those spending extended hours at their desks. Here's how to address frequent ergonomic problems effectively:

1. **Lower Back Pain**: Lower back pain often results from poor lumbar support or lack of movement. Solution: Adjust lumbar support, use a pillow if necessary, and practice regular core-strengthening exercises.
2. **Neck and Shoulder Pain**: This pain typically comes from monitor positioning or hunching. Solution: Ensure your monitor is at eye level, take regular neck and shoulder stretches, and avoid leaning forward.
3. **Wrist and Hand Discomfort**: Wrist pain is often due to improper keyboard and mouse placement. Solution: Keep wrists in a neutral position, use a wrist rest, and avoid overextending when reaching for the mouse.
4. **Eye Strain and Headaches**: Eye strain can stem from screen glare or improper brightness. Solution: Adjust screen brightness, position the monitor to avoid glare, and follow the 20-20-20 rule (look at something 20 feet away for 20 seconds every 20 minutes).

Integrating Movement into an Ergonomic Workspace

Even a well-designed ergonomic workspace cannot fully mitigate the impact of prolonged sitting. Integrating movement into your work routine is essential for reducing muscle fatigue, improving circulation, and maintaining alertness throughout the day. Here are several practical strategies for incorporating movement:

1. **Micro-Breaks**: Take short breaks every 30-45 minutes to stand, stretch, or walk around. Set reminders to encourage consistent movement throughout the day.
2. **Desk Stretches and Exercises**: Engage in simple exercises such as shoulder shrugs, wrist stretches, seated leg lifts, and neck rolls. These exercises prevent stiffness and promote flexibility without interrupting productivity.
3. **Standing Desk or Desk Converter**: Alternate between sitting and standing to prevent prolonged strain. Using a standing desk or desk converter provides flexibility and reduces the negative effects of sitting.
4. **Walking Meetings**: For discussions or brainstorming sessions that don't require a screen, suggest a walking meeting. Walking stimulates creativity, encourages movement, and provides a break from the static desk setup.
5. **Stretching Routine**: Set aside time for a quick stretching routine during lunch or after work. Target areas prone to stiffness, like the neck, shoulders, lower back, and hips, to release tension and increase mobility.

Long-Term Benefits of an Ergonomic Workspace

Investing time and effort in creating an ergonomic workspace can lead to numerous long-term benefits, enhancing not only physical well-being but also mental health and work satisfaction:

1. **Reduced Risk of Injury and Chronic Pain**: Proper ergonomics prevent repetitive strain injuries and reduce the likelihood of developing chronic conditions like lower back pain, carpal tunnel syndrome, and shoulder impingement.
2. **Enhanced Focus and Efficiency**: When physical discomfort is minimized, employees can maintain focus for longer periods, leading to higher productivity, fewer mistakes, and better overall performance.

3. **Improved Job Satisfaction**: An ergonomic environment demonstrates a commitment to employee well-being, fostering a positive workplace culture that prioritizes comfort and health.
4. **Better Work-Life Balance**: Employees who work in ergonomic environments are less likely to take time off due to pain or discomfort, contributing to a better balance between work demands and personal life.

Creating an Ergonomic Workspace on a Budget

While some ergonomic equipment can be costly, there are many low-cost options and DIY solutions that make an ergonomic workspace accessible. Here are some affordable ways to improve your workstation ergonomics:

1. **Use a Rolled Towel for Lumbar Support**: If your chair lacks built-in lumbar support, a small pillow or rolled towel can provide similar benefits.
2. **Raise Your Monitor**: Books, shoeboxes, or monitor risers can be used to adjust the height of your screen to eye level, reducing neck strain without the need for expensive adjustable monitor arms.
3. **Keyboard and Mouse Pads with Wrist Support**: Inexpensive wrist supports help maintain neutral wrist positioning, reducing the risk of strain.
4. **Lighting Adjustments**: Use a simple desk lamp with an adjustable brightness setting to reduce eye strain. Blue light screen protectors are also affordable solutions to help prevent digital eye strain.

An ergonomic workspace is a vital component of a healthy and productive work environment. By making adjustments to support proper posture, reduce strain, and encourage movement, you can prevent common workplace injuries and maintain physical and mental well-being. Ergonomics isn't just about reducing discomfort; it's a proactive approach to fostering a sustainable, fulfilling work life.

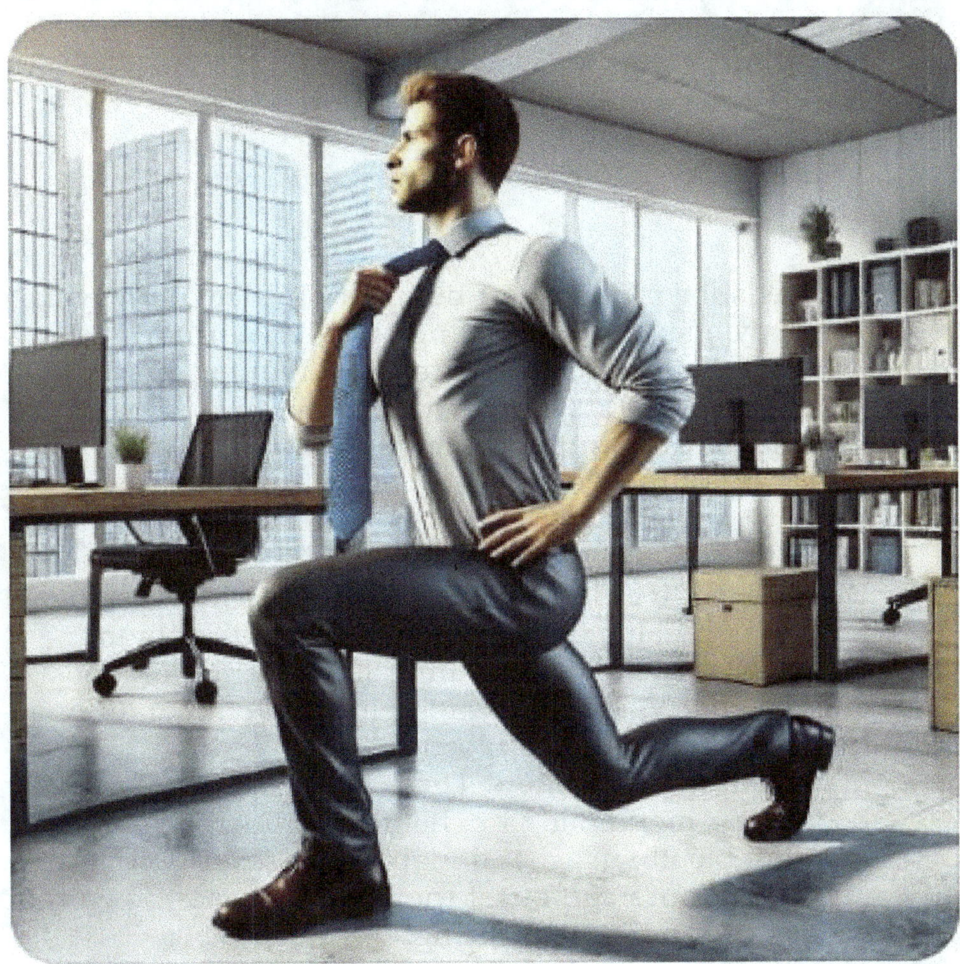

Chapter 4: Micro Workouts for Busy Professionals

In a fast-paced world where work demands often leave little time for traditional workouts, micro workouts offer an effective way to stay fit and energized. Micro workouts are short, targeted bursts of physical activity that can be performed in just a few minutes without disrupting your workday. These small, consistent movements can be just as beneficial as longer workouts, helping to boost circulation, improve mental clarity, and reduce the negative effects of prolonged sitting.

In this chapter, we'll dive deeper into the science behind micro workouts, explore practical exercises for different parts of the body, and look at strategies to build a consistent, energizing routine that keeps you active and engaged—even on the busiest of days.

The Science of Micro Workouts: Maximizing Impact in Minimal Time

Research has shown that short bouts of physical activity can be surprisingly effective at boosting overall health and wellness. The human body benefits from frequent movement, and regular, small bursts of activity can improve cardiovascular health, support mental well-being, and counteract the stiffness and fatigue associated with long periods of sitting.

1. **Enhanced Circulation**: Micro workouts increase blood flow, which helps deliver oxygen and nutrients to muscles and vital organs. Improved circulation boosts energy, sharpens focus, and helps prevent conditions like varicose veins and blood clots.
2. **Metabolism Activation**: These short bursts of activity boost your metabolic rate, helping to burn calories, regulate blood sugar, and maintain a healthy weight. Micro workouts can offset the metabolic slowdown that occurs with prolonged sitting.
3. **Mental Rejuvenation**: Physical activity stimulates the release of endorphins, which alleviate stress and improve mood. Micro workouts offer a quick mental reset, reducing stress and enhancing cognitive performance.
4. **Muscle Engagement**: Regular micro workouts engage muscles that may otherwise become inactive during a typical workday. Keeping muscles activated prevents tension, reduces the risk of repetitive strain injuries, and supports overall strength.
5. **Combating Sedentary Behavior**: Even a few minutes of movement each hour can help combat the negative effects of sedentary behavior, improving cardiovascular health, strengthening muscles, and supporting long-term wellness.

To make the most of micro workouts, it's essential to target areas most affected by sitting and sedentary behavior. A balanced micro workout routine includes exercises that strengthen, stretch, and mobilize key muscles, including the core, legs, back, shoulders, and neck.

1. **Core Strength**: A strong core supports posture, reduces lower back strain, and improves overall stability. Core-focused exercises can be discreetly done while sitting or standing at your desk.
2. **Upper Body Mobility**: Shoulders, upper back, and arms often carry tension from typing and screen use. Mobility exercises for these areas alleviate tightness, support posture, and prevent repetitive strain.
3. **Lower Body Strength and Flexibility**: Sitting weakens the legs, hips, and glutes and reduces circulation. Targeted lower body exercises maintain strength, improve circulation, and reduce stiffness in these areas.
4. **Joint Flexibility and Mobility**: Regular joint mobility exercises reduce stiffness, enhance range of motion, and prevent injuries. These exercises benefit commonly strained joints, including the neck, shoulders, wrists, and ankles.

Desk-Friendly Micro Workouts: Effective Exercises to Stay Active

Here are some practical micro workout exercises that can be easily done at your desk or workspace. Each exercise takes only a few minutes and can be performed multiple times a day to keep your body moving and engaged.

Seated Tummy Tucks

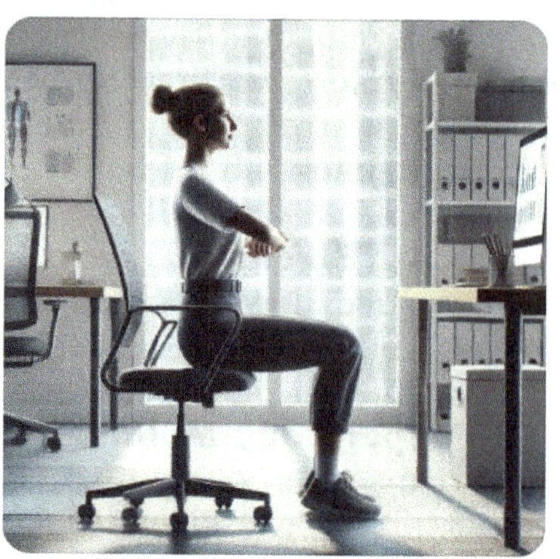

- Sit upright in your chair, engage your core by pulling your belly button toward your spine, and hold for a few seconds.
- Release and repeat 10-15 times. This exercise strengthens the core and improves posture without requiring noticeable movement.

Standing Oblique Crunches

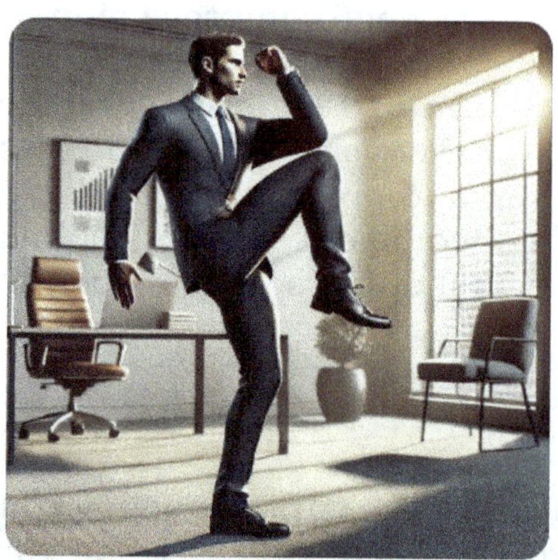

- Stand next to your desk, place your hands on your hips, and lift one knee while bringing the opposite elbow toward it.
- Alternate sides, performing 10-15 reps on each side. This exercise targets the obliques and strengthens the core.

Seated Bicycle Crunches

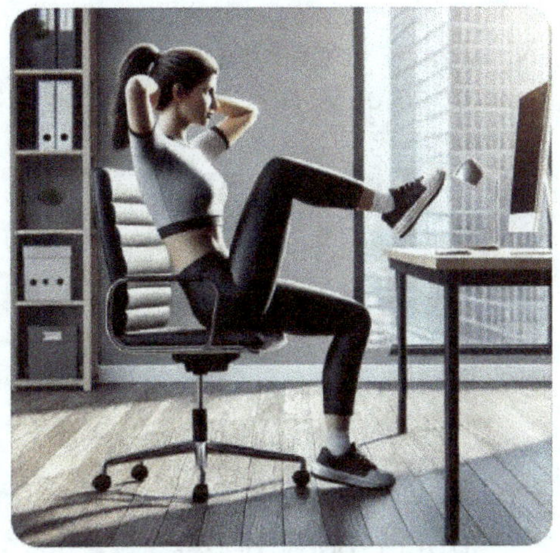

- Sit at the edge of your chair, with hands behind your head.
- Lift one knee toward your chest and twist your opposite elbow toward it, then switch sides, mimicking a "bicycle" motion.
- Perform 10-15 reps per side. This move engages the core and promotes spinal mobility.

2. Upper Body and Shoulder Mobility Exercises

Shoulder Blade Squeezes

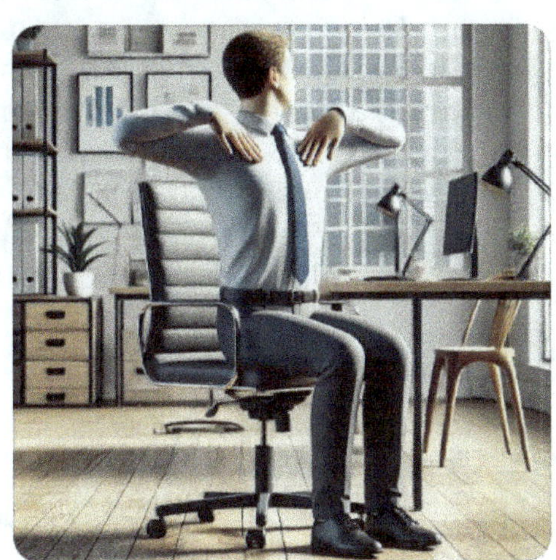

- Sit or stand up straight with your arms at your sides.
- Squeeze your shoulder blades together, hold for a few seconds, and release.
- Repeat 10-15 times. This exercise strengthens the upper back and reduces shoulder tension.

Desk Dips

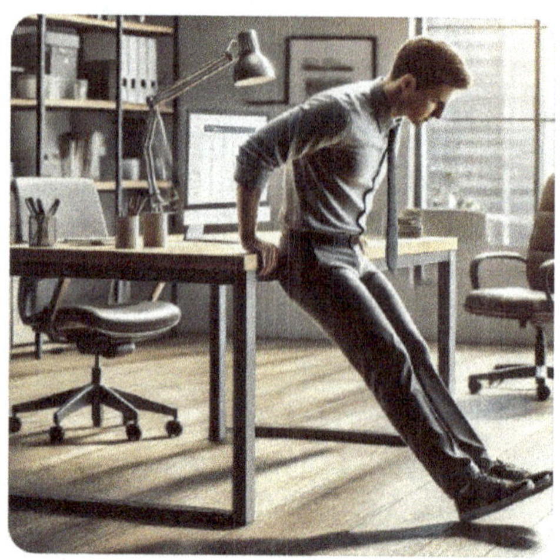

- Place your hands on the edge of your desk, palms facing down, and walk your feet forward to form a 45-degree angle.
- Bend your elbows to lower your body, then push back up.
- Perform 10-15 reps. Desk dips strengthen the triceps and engage the shoulders, giving an upper-body boost.

Wall Angels

- Stand with your back against a wall, arms at a 90-degree angle.
- Slowly slide your arms up and down against the wall as if doing a "snow angel" motion.
- Perform 10-15 reps. Wall angels improve shoulder flexibility and help correct posture.

3. Lower Body Strength and Circulation Exercises

Chair Squats

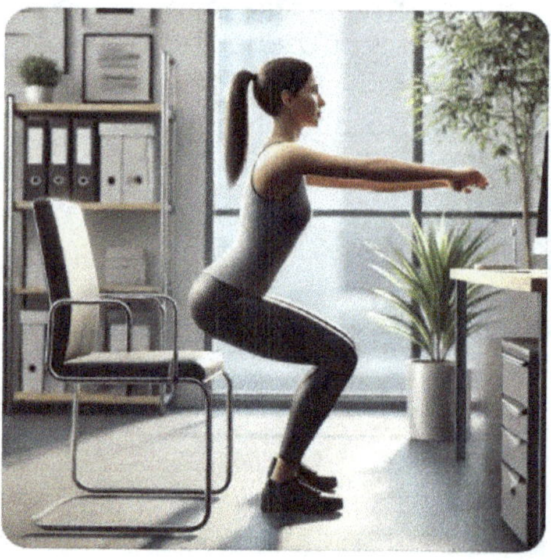

- Stand in front of your chair, feet hip-width apart.
- Lower yourself toward the chair as if you're about to sit, but stop just before touching and rise back up.
- Repeat 10-15 times. This exercise strengthens the legs and glutes and promotes circulation.

Calf Raises

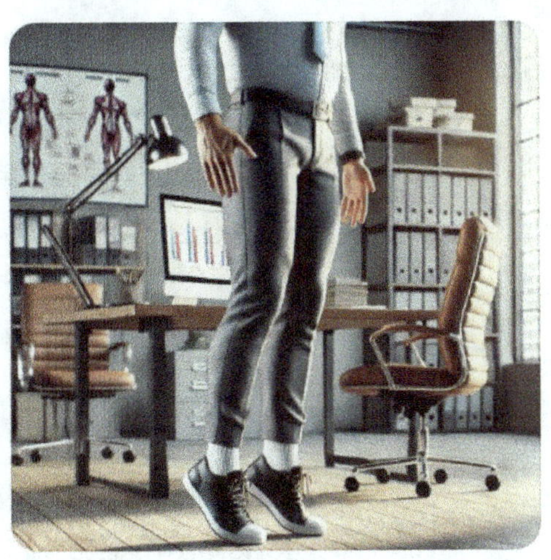

- Stand with feet hip-width apart, holding onto your desk for balance if needed.
- Rise onto the balls of your feet, hold for a few seconds, and lower back down.
- Repeat 15-20 times. Calf raises improve circulation and strengthen the lower legs.

Desk Lunges

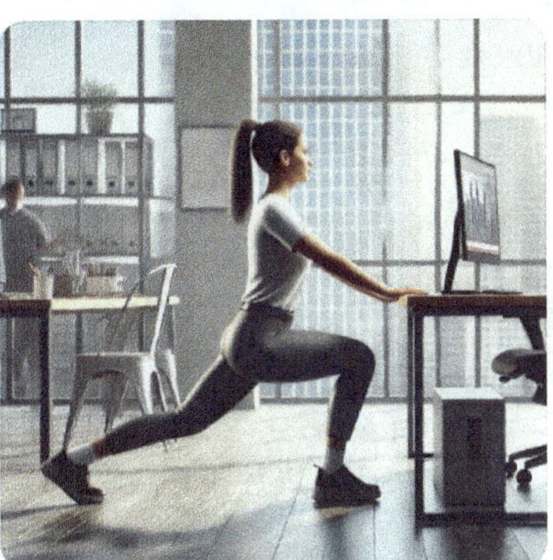

- Stand with one leg forward and the other back, hands resting on the desk for balance.
- Lower into a lunge, bending both knees, and push back up.
- Alternate legs, performing 10-15 reps per side. Desk lunges engage the legs, glutes, and core.

Seated Hamstring Stretch

- Sit at the edge of your chair and extend one leg out, keeping the heel on the floor and toes pointing up.
- Lean forward slightly, reaching toward your toes.
- Hold for 15-30 seconds per leg. This stretch releases tension in the hamstrings and lower back.

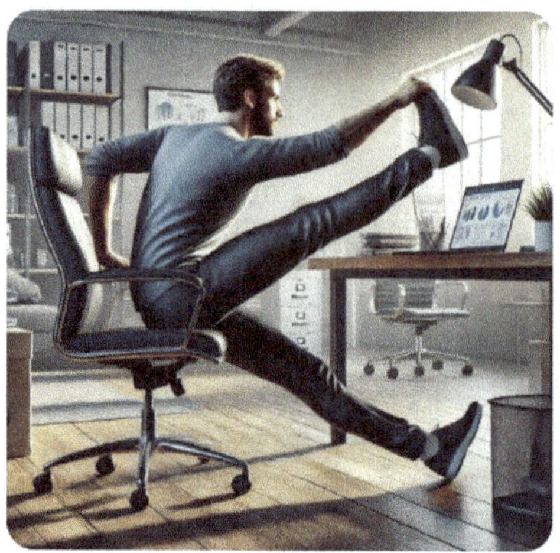

Wrist Flexor Stretch

- Extend one arm in front of you, with your palm facing up.
- Use your opposite hand to gently pull back on the fingers, stretching the wrist and forearm.
- Hold for 15-30 seconds on each side. This stretch alleviates tension in the wrists from typing.
- Perform this stretch with both the palms facing up and the palms facing down.

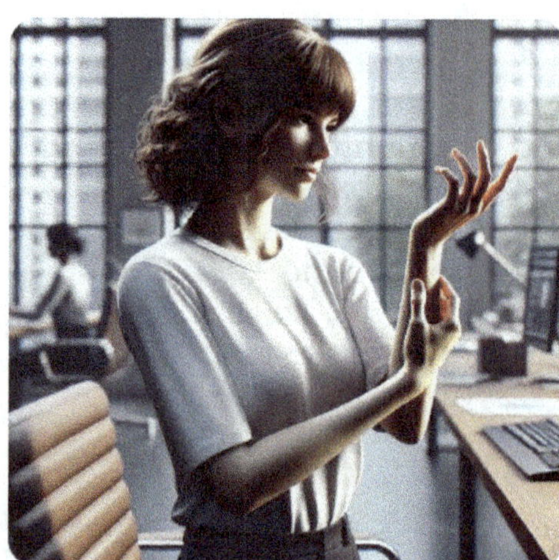

Ankle Circles

- While seated, lift one foot off the ground and rotate your ankle in a circular motion.
- Perform 10-15 circles in each direction, then switch feet. Ankle circles improve joint mobility and promote lower leg circulation.

Building a micro workout routine into your day doesn't require a complete schedule overhaul. Small breaks for movement can easily fit between tasks, meetings, and emails. Here's a sample routine to help guide you:

1. **Morning Activation**: Start your day with shoulder blade squeezes, calf raises, and seated tummy tucks to energize your muscles and prepare for a productive morning.
2. **Mid-Morning Stretch**: After a couple of hours of desk work, perform standing oblique crunches, wall angels, and ankle circles to refresh your body and keep energy levels up.
3. **Lunchtime Power Moves**: During part of your lunch break, try chair squats, desk lunges, and seated hamstring stretches to boost circulation, release tension, and recharge for the afternoon.
4. **Afternoon Re-Energizer**: During the afternoon slump, do desk dips, wrist flexor stretches, and seated bicycle crunches to shake off fatigue and maintain mental clarity.
5. **End-of-Day Release**: Finish your workday with a set of neck stretches, seated forward folds, and shoulder rolls to release any lingering tension and transition smoothly into your evening.

The Benefits of Micro Workouts Beyond Physical Fitness

The advantages of micro workouts extend beyond physical benefits; they positively impact mental well-being and overall work performance.

1. **Improved Focus and Productivity**: Physical activity increases blood flow to the brain, which improves focus, memory, and problem-solving abilities. These quick exercises can reduce mental fatigue and keep you alert throughout the day.

2. **Reduced Work-Related Stress**: Movement encourages the release of endorphins, helping to reduce stress, elevate mood, and improve resilience to challenges. Micro workouts provide a brief mental break that can alleviate work-related stress and improve overall job satisfaction.

3. **Long-Term Wellness**: Regular movement throughout the day can help prevent lifestyle-related health conditions, such as obesity, diabetes, and cardiovascular disease. Micro workouts also support joint health and mobility, which are essential for maintaining long-term physical function.

4. **Increased Confidence and Mental Clarity**: Achieving small goals, like completing a set of desk exercises, can boost self-confidence and provide a sense of accomplishment. The clarity gained from short workouts often spills over into improved decision-making and creativity.

Staying Consistent with Micro Workouts: Tips for Long-Term Success

Building a habit of micro workouts requires consistency and a few reminders to keep you on track. Here are some tips to make micro workouts a lasting part of your daily routine:

1. **Set Timers**: Use reminders on your phone or computer to alert you every hour or two to get up, stretch, or perform a quick workout. This helps you build movement into your routine without needing to remember.

2. **Use Movement Apps**: Many fitness apps offer short workout routines or timed reminders to get up and move. These apps can guide you through micro workouts and help you stay on track.

3. **Find a Workout Buddy**: If possible, recruit a colleague or friend to join you in your micro workout routine. This can add a social aspect and keep you accountable.

4. **Focus on Variety**: Rotate between different exercises to keep your routine interesting and avoid fatigue. Variety also ensures that you target multiple muscle groups and prevent repetitive strain.
5. **Celebrate Small Wins**: Acknowledge each completed set of exercises as a win, whether it's a set of desk push-ups or a quick stretching break. Celebrating small victories reinforces positive behavior and builds motivation.

Micro workouts are a powerful tool for improving physical and mental health in a busy work environment. By incorporating short, targeted exercises into your day, you can combat the effects of prolonged sitting, reduce stress, and enhance your focus and productivity. Remember that every small movement counts, and consistent micro workouts contribute to long-term wellness and vitality.

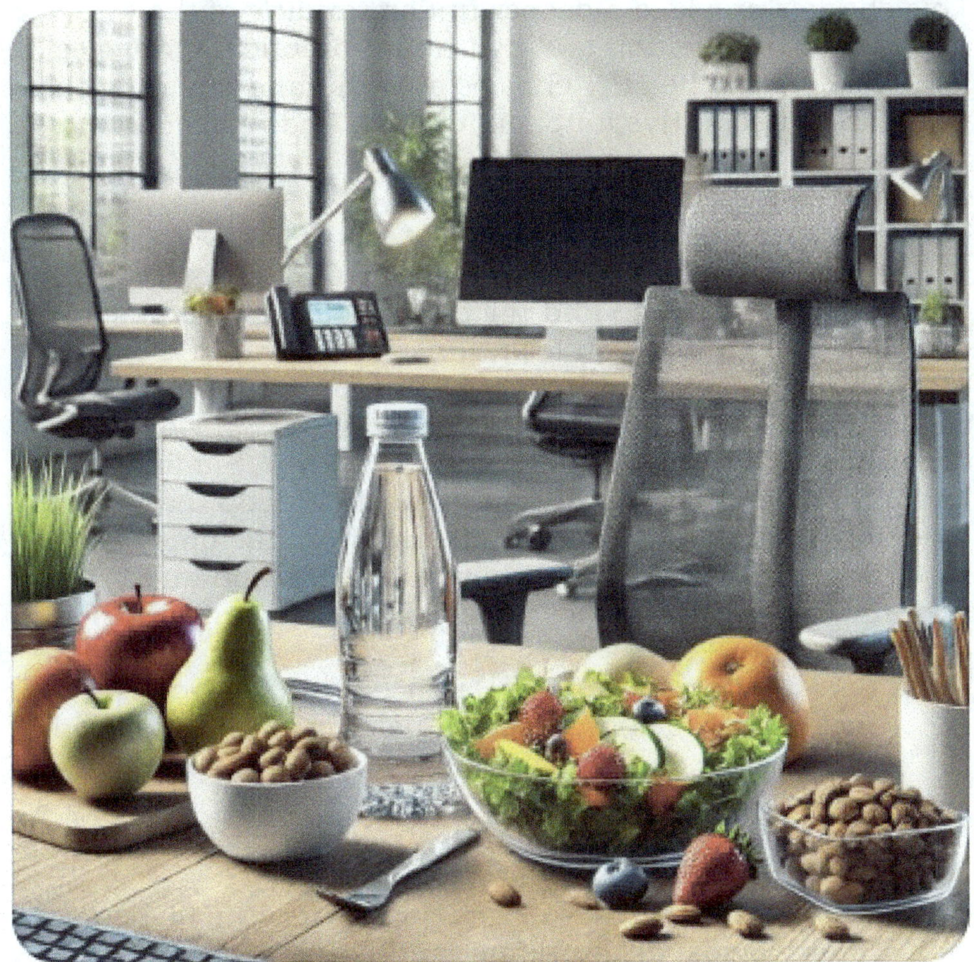

Chapter 5: Nutrition and Hydration at Work

A balanced diet and proper hydration are crucial for maintaining energy, focus, and resilience throughout the workday. Unfortunately, the fast-paced nature of modern workplaces often leads employees to rely on convenience foods, caffeine, and vending machine snacks, which can lead to energy crashes, reduced productivity, and long-term health challenges. By prioritizing nutrient-dense foods and adequate hydration, you can fuel your body and mind for peak performance, supporting both short-term productivity and long-term health.

This chapter provides a deeper understanding of the importance of nutrition and hydration, practical strategies for incorporating healthy choices at work, and key nutrients that support cognitive function, energy, and resilience against stress.

Why Nutrition and Hydration Matter in the Workplace

Food is the body's fuel, and the quality of that fuel has a direct impact on how you feel, think, and perform. Poor dietary choices can lead to energy slumps, irritability, and reduced focus, while healthy, balanced foods provide consistent energy and support mental clarity. Similarly, hydration is critical to brain and muscle function, and even mild dehydration can impair concentration, memory, and mood. Here's a closer look at how good nutrition and hydration positively impact workplace performance:

1. **Steady Energy Levels**: Balanced, nutrient-dense meals release energy slowly, helping you avoid blood sugar spikes and crashes that lead to fatigue. Choosing foods rich in protein, fiber, and healthy fats sustains energy levels and helps you stay productive throughout the day.
2. **Enhanced Cognitive Function**: Nutrients like omega-3 fatty acids, antioxidants, and B vitamins support brain health, improving memory, concentration, and problem-solving abilities. Consistently fueling the brain with these nutrients helps you stay sharp, make better decisions, and respond effectively to workplace challenges.
3. **Stress Management and Emotional Stability**: Nutrient-rich foods support the body's ability to handle stress. For example, complex carbohydrates and magnesium promote the production of serotonin, a mood-regulating neurotransmitter, while vitamin C and B vitamins support the nervous system's stress response.
4. **Immune Function and Overall Health**: A healthy diet strengthens the immune system, reducing the risk of

illness and absenteeism. Nutrient-dense foods rich in vitamins C, D, and zinc enhance immune function, while a balanced diet supports resilience against infections.

5. **Physical Comfort and Joint Health**: Hydration and anti-inflammatory foods help reduce physical discomfort from prolonged sitting, like joint stiffness and muscle aches. Proper hydration also prevents issues like dry eyes and headaches, common among people who work on screens.

Water is essential for every cell, tissue, and organ in the body. Yet, it's easy to overlook hydration during a busy workday, especially when caffeinated drinks and sugary beverages are available. Even slight dehydration can impair cognitive function, energy, and mood, affecting overall productivity and well-being. Here's why hydration is critical for workplace performance:

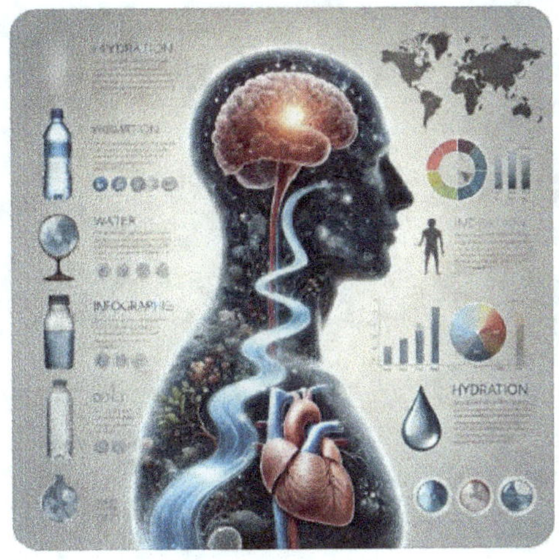

1. **Brain Function and Focus**: The brain relies on water to maintain focus, memory, and cognitive processing. Dehydration can cause brain cells to shrink slightly, leading to poor concentration, mental fatigue, and even short-term memory lapses.

2. **Energy and Metabolic Support**: Water is essential for converting food into energy and transporting oxygen and nutrients throughout the body. Dehydration slows down these processes, resulting in lower energy levels and reduced physical endurance.

3. **Mood Regulation and Stress Resilience**: Hydration plays a role in regulating cortisol, the body's main stress hormone. Staying hydrated helps maintain a stable mood and reduces the effects of stress, keeping you calm and focused during challenging tasks.

4. **Physical Comfort and Mobility**: Water lubricates joints, which helps prevent stiffness and discomfort, especially if you're sitting for long periods. Hydration also helps alleviate dry eyes, a common complaint among those who work in air-conditioned offices or spend long hours at a computer.

Building a Balanced Workplace Diet: Key Strategies

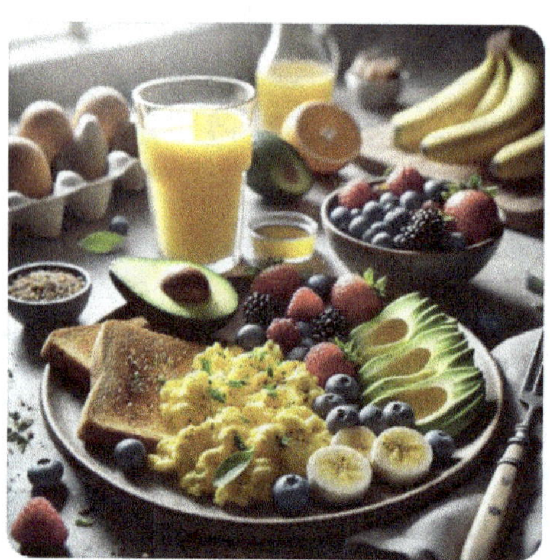

Healthy eating in the workplace doesn't have to be complicated. With some planning and simple adjustments, you can create a daily meal and snack routine that supports energy, focus, and well-being. Here are some practical strategies for building a balanced diet at work:

1. Start with a Power-Packed Breakfast

A nutritious breakfast is essential for kickstarting your metabolism, fueling your body, and setting a positive tone for the rest of your day. Skipping breakfast or opting for high-sugar, processed foods can lead to energy crashes, irritability, and reduced mental clarity by mid-morning. Instead, focus on a balanced breakfast that includes complex carbohydrates, healthy fats, and protein to provide lasting energy, improve focus, and enhance mood.

Eating a balanced breakfast has numerous benefits that extend beyond just providing energy:

1. **Sustained Energy Levels**: Foods rich in complex carbohydrates, like oats and whole grains, release energy slowly, keeping your blood sugar stable and helping you avoid the mid-morning slump.
2. **Enhanced Cognitive Function**: A balanced breakfast supports brain health, improving memory, focus, and decision-making. Protein and healthy fats help stabilize blood sugar, ensuring your brain has a steady supply of glucose.
3. **Improved Mood and Stress Management**: Foods with healthy fats and complex carbs promote the release of serotonin, a neurotransmitter that helps regulate mood and stress response, keeping you calm and focused.
4. **Reduced Cravings and Better Food Choices**: Eating a satisfying breakfast reduces the likelihood of reaching for unhealthy snacks later. Protein and fiber help you feel full, preventing hunger-driven decisions that can derail healthy eating goals.

Key Components of a Power-Packed Breakfast

A power-packed breakfast includes three primary components: complex carbohydrates, protein, and healthy fats. This combination provides a balanced release of energy and supports brain and body function throughout the morning.

1. **Complex Carbohydrates**: These carbs provide a steady source of energy, as they break down slowly and prevent blood sugar spikes. Examples include whole grains, fruits, and vegetables.
2. **Protein**: Protein is essential for muscle repair, immune function, and maintaining stable blood sugar levels. It also helps you feel full and satisfied, reducing

hunger later in the day. Good sources include eggs, Greek yogurt, cottage cheese, and plant-based options like tofu or legumes.
3. **Healthy Fats**: Healthy fats, like those found in nuts, seeds, avocados, and olive oil, support brain health, hormone balance, and long-lasting energy. Including fats in your breakfast helps you stay satisfied and enhances the absorption of fat-soluble vitamins like A, D, E, and K.

Breakfast Ideas for a Power-Packed Start

Here are some balanced breakfast ideas that are easy to prepare, nutrient-dense, and convenient for busy mornings:

1. Overnight Oats

Overnight oats are an easy, make-ahead option that provides a blend of fiber, protein, and healthy fats:

- **Ingredients**: ½ cup rolled oats, 1 cup milk or dairy-free alternative, 1 tablespoon chia seeds, a handful of berries, and a sprinkle of nuts or seeds.
- **Preparation**: Combine all ingredients in a jar or container, stir well, and refrigerate overnight. In the morning, add additional toppings like a drizzle of almond butter or sliced banana for extra flavor and nutrients.

Why It Works: This meal is high in fiber and protein, thanks to oats and chia seeds, while the berries add antioxidants, and the nuts or seeds provide healthy fats.

2. Greek Yogurt Parfait with Nuts and Berries

This quick option is packed with protein, fiber, and healthy fats:

- **Ingredients**: 1 cup Greek yogurt, ¼ cup fresh berries, 1 tablespoon nuts or seeds, and a drizzle of honey or a sprinkle of cinnamon.

- **Preparation**: Layer Greek yogurt with berries and top with nuts or seeds. You can add honey or cinnamon for a touch of sweetness and flavor.

Why It Works: Greek yogurt is high in protein, which promotes satiety, while berries add vitamins and antioxidants. Nuts and seeds provide fiber and healthy fats, which help keep energy levels steady.

3. Avocado Toast with Eggs

Avocado toast is a satisfying, nutrient-dense breakfast that includes complex carbs, protein, and healthy fats:

- **Ingredients**: 1 slice of whole-grain bread, ½ avocado, 1-2 eggs (poached, scrambled, or fried), and a pinch of salt, pepper, or red pepper flakes.
- **Preparation**: Toast the bread, spread mashed avocado on top, and add the eggs. Sprinkle with seasoning of choice.

Why It Works: Whole-grain toast provides complex carbs for steady energy, while avocado adds heart-healthy fats and fiber. Eggs contribute protein, making this meal both filling and energizing.

4. Smoothie with Protein, Greens, and Healthy Fats

A smoothie is a convenient option for those with busy schedules, and it's easy to customize to meet your nutritional needs:

- **Ingredients**: 1 cup almond milk or dairy milk, a handful of spinach, 1 banana or ½ cup berries, 1 tablespoon chia seeds or ground flaxseed, and a scoop of protein powder (optional).
- **Preparation**: Blend all ingredients until smooth. Add ice for a thicker texture if desired.

Why It Works: This smoothie includes complex carbs (from fruit), protein, and healthy fats (from chia or flax seeds). Leafy greens add fiber, antioxidants, and essential vitamins.

5. Veggie Omelette with Whole-Grain Toast

An omelette packed with vegetables and served with whole-grain toast provides a balanced mix of protein, fiber, and vitamins:

- **Ingredients**: 2 eggs, a handful of spinach, diced bell peppers, and tomatoes, 1 slice of whole-grain toast.
- **Preparation**: Whisk eggs, pour them into a hot pan, and add the vegetables. Cook until eggs are set, then serve with whole-grain toast on the side.

Why It Works: Eggs provide high-quality protein, while vegetables add fiber, vitamins, and minerals. Whole-grain toast completes the meal with complex carbs for long-lasting energy.

Tips for Making Breakfast Part of Your Routine

If mornings are rushed, it can be challenging to fit in a healthy breakfast. Here are some tips to ensure you start your day with a nutritious meal, even on busy mornings:

1. **Prep Ahead**: Prepare breakfast the night before, especially if you're opting for meals like overnight oats or yogurt parfaits. This way, all you need to do in the morning is grab and go.
2. **Set a Routine**: Establish a morning routine that includes time for breakfast. Prioritizing breakfast, even if it's quick, helps prevent unhealthy snacking later in the day.
3. **Use Portable Options**: If you don't have time to eat breakfast at home, choose portable options like smoothies, protein bars, or breakfast wraps that can be eaten on your commute or once you arrive at work.
4. **Incorporate Variety**: Vary your breakfast choices to keep things interesting and ensure you're getting a range of nutrients. Rotating through different breakfasts also helps prevent "flavor fatigue."
5. **Consider a High-Protein Option for Sustained Energy**: If you're especially prone to mid-morning

hunger, choose breakfasts that are higher in protein, as they can help you feel fuller for longer.

Breakfast Boosters: Nutrient-Dense Add-Ins

To maximize the nutritional value of your breakfast, consider adding some of these nutrient-dense ingredients. They're easy to incorporate and offer a variety of health benefits:

1. **Chia Seeds**: High in fiber, protein, and omega-3s, chia seeds promote satiety, support brain health, and provide lasting energy. Add a tablespoon to smoothies, yogurt, or oats.
2. **Ground Flaxseed**: Another excellent source of fiber and omega-3s, flaxseed supports heart health and digestion. Sprinkle a tablespoon over yogurt, oatmeal, or blend it into smoothies.
3. **Nut Butters**: Almond, peanut, and cashew butters are rich in healthy fats, protein, and essential minerals like magnesium. Adding a small amount to toast, oatmeal, or smoothies can help stabilize blood sugar and keep you satisfied.
4. **Leafy Greens**: Spinach, kale, and other greens are low in calories but packed with vitamins, minerals, and antioxidants. Add a handful to your smoothie or omelette for an extra nutrient boost.
5. **Berries**: Blueberries, strawberries, and raspberries are high in antioxidants, fiber, and vitamin C. They can be added to almost any breakfast to enhance flavor and add a nutritional boost.
6. **Greek Yogurt**: A high-protein, probiotic-rich food, Greek yogurt supports digestion, boosts immune function, and provides a creamy texture to smoothies and parfaits.

Avoiding Common Breakfast Pitfalls

While breakfast offers a fantastic opportunity to fuel your day, some choices can work against you, causing energy crashes and hunger soon after eating. Here are some breakfast pitfalls to avoid:

1. **Sugary Cereals and Pastries**: These foods cause rapid spikes and drops in blood sugar, leading to energy crashes and mid-morning cravings. Instead, opt for whole grains or oats for steady energy.
2. **Skipping Protein**: Many breakfasts are carb-heavy without enough protein, which can lead to quick hunger and reduced mental clarity. Always include a protein source to keep you full and focused.
3. **Processed Breakfast Bars**: Many breakfast bars are high in sugar and low in nutrients. If you choose a bar, look for one with at least 8-10 grams of protein and minimal added sugar.
4. **Relying on Only Caffeine**: Coffee alone can boost alertness, but it doesn't provide lasting energy. Pair your morning coffee with a balanced meal to prevent caffeine-induced crashes.

The Long-Term Benefits of a Power-Packed Breakfast

By consistently starting your day with a nutritious breakfast, you lay the groundwork for optimal mental and physical performance. Some of the long-term benefits include:

1. **Increased Productivity**: A balanced breakfast enhances focus and concentration, allowing you to tackle complex tasks with greater ease.
2. **Improved Mood and Stress Resilience**: A satisfying breakfast helps stabilize blood sugar and supports the production of mood-boosting neurotransmitters, reducing irritability and enhancing emotional resilience.
3. **Better Weight Management**: Eating a filling, nutrient-dense breakfast reduces the likelihood of overeating later in the day and helps regulate appetite.
4. **Enhanced Long-Term Health**: Regularly consuming a balanced breakfast supports heart health, maintains

steady blood sugar, and reduces the risk of chronic conditions such as diabetes and obesity.

2. Pack a Balanced Lunch to Prevent Afternoon Slumps

Lunch should be filling but not so heavy that it causes fatigue. Aim for a mix of lean protein, fiber, and healthy fats to provide sustained energy and prevent the post-lunch crash. Here are some balanced lunch ideas that are easy to prepare and bring to work:

- **Quinoa Salad with Grilled Chicken and Vegetables**: Combine quinoa, grilled chicken, mixed vegetables, and a drizzle of olive oil for a balanced, satisfying meal.
- **Wraps with Protein and Veggies**: Use a whole-grain wrap filled with lean protein (such as turkey, chicken, or tofu), plenty of veggies, and a spread like hummus or avocado for added healthy fats.
- **Chickpea and Spinach Salad with Feta**: A hearty salad with chickpeas, spinach, feta cheese, and a handful of nuts offers fiber, protein, and essential nutrients.

3. Choose Smart Snacks for Consistent Energy

Healthy snacks help keep blood sugar stable and prevent the urge to reach for sugary treats. Opt for snacks that provide a mix of protein, fiber, and healthy fats for long-lasting energy. Here are some nutritious snack ideas that are easy to pack and eat at your desk:

- **Nut Butter and Apple Slices**: Pair apple slices with almond or peanut butter for a snack rich in fiber, vitamins, and healthy fats.
- **Greek Yogurt with Berries**: Greek yogurt provides protein, while berries add antioxidants and natural sweetness.
- **Veggies and Hummus**: Carrot, cucumber, and bell pepper sticks with hummus offer a combination of fiber, vitamins, and plant-based protein.
- **Trail Mix with Nuts and Dark Chocolate**: A small handful of trail mix with unsalted nuts and a few pieces of dark chocolate provides a nutrient-dense snack and satisfies sweet cravings.

4. Limit Processed Foods and Sugary Beverages

Processed foods and sugary snacks may offer a quick energy boost, but they often lead to energy crashes that affect productivity. To avoid these fluctuations, focus on whole foods that release energy gradually. If you're craving something sweet, reach for fruit or a small piece of dark chocolate for a healthier alternative.

Maintaining Hydration Throughout the Workday

Drinking enough water is essential, but it can be easy to forget during a busy day. These simple strategies can help you stay hydrated without much effort:

1. Keep a Water Bottle at Your Desk

Having a reusable water bottle within arm's reach serves as a reminder to drink water regularly. Set goals to drink a certain number of refills each day, or use a larger bottle if it encourages you to drink more at once.

2. Infuse Water with Natural Flavors

If plain water doesn't appeal to you, try infusing it with fruits like lemon, cucumber, or berries, or add herbs like mint. Infused water is refreshing, and it may encourage you to drink more throughout the day.

3. Use Hydration Reminders

Set reminders on your phone or computer to prompt you to drink water every hour. Many apps also track water intake and send reminders, helping you meet your hydration goals.

4. Supplement with Water-Rich Foods

In addition to drinking water, include water-rich foods in your diet, such as cucumbers, oranges, tomatoes, and leafy greens. These foods contribute to your overall hydration and are also packed with vitamins and antioxidants.

Key Nutrients to Support Cognitive Function, Energy, and Mood

Certain nutrients are particularly beneficial for workplace performance, supporting cognitive function, energy, and emotional resilience. Here are some key nutrients and food sources to include in your workday diet:

1. **B Vitamins**: Essential for energy production and brain health. Foods rich in B vitamins include whole grains, leafy greens, eggs, and lean meats.
2. **Omega-3 Fatty Acids**: Omega-3s support brain function, memory, and mood regulation. Sources include fatty fish (like salmon and sardines), walnuts, chia seeds, and flaxseeds.
3. **Magnesium**: This mineral helps with muscle relaxation, stress management, and energy production. Foods rich in magnesium include spinach, almonds, pumpkin seeds, and whole grains.
4. **Iron**: Iron is vital for oxygen transport, energy, and concentration. Low iron levels can lead to fatigue and brain fog. Iron-rich foods include red meat, beans, lentils, and spinach.
5. **Antioxidants**: Antioxidants protect brain cells from damage, supporting cognitive function and overall health. Berries, dark chocolate, nuts, and green tea are rich in antioxidants.
6. **Vitamin D**: Important for mood regulation, immune function, and overall energy. While it's challenging to get enough vitamin D from food alone, foods like fatty fish, fortified milk, and eggs can contribute to your intake. Additionally, spending a few minutes outdoors can help boost your vitamin D levels.

To put these strategies into practice, here's a sample meal and snack plan designed to sustain energy, focus, and productivity throughout the day:

- **Breakfast**: Overnight oats with chia seeds, berries, and a sprinkle of walnuts. Provides fiber, protein, and healthy fats to start the day with sustained energy.
- **Mid-Morning Snack**: Greek yogurt with mixed berries. A source of protein, antioxidants, and natural sweetness for a morning boost.
- **Lunch**: Grain bowl with quinoa, grilled chicken, mixed greens, roasted vegetables, and avocado. This balanced meal supplies protein, fiber, vitamins, and healthy fats for a filling, energizing lunch.
- **Afternoon Snack**: Carrot and celery sticks with hummus. Offers fiber, vitamins, and plant-based protein to stave off afternoon hunger.
- **Dinner**: Baked salmon with steamed broccoli, a sweet potato, and a side salad with olive oil dressing. Rich in omega-3 fatty acids, fiber, and vitamins to replenish nutrients and support mental and physical recovery after the workday.

Long-Term Benefits of Prioritizing Workplace Nutrition and Hydration

When you consistently fuel your body with balanced nutrition and stay hydrated, you experience both immediate and long-term benefits:

1. **Improved Focus and Mental Clarity**: A nutrient-dense diet and proper hydration enhance cognitive function, memory, and focus, making it easier to complete complex tasks and stay on top of work demands.
2. **Steady Energy Levels**: Balanced meals and snacks provide a consistent release of energy, helping you

avoid the highs and lows that come from caffeine and sugar.

3. **Enhanced Stress Management**: Nutrients that support the nervous system, such as magnesium and B vitamins, improve your body's ability to cope with stress, reducing anxiety and improving resilience.
4. **Stronger Immune Function**: A healthy diet strengthens the immune system, reducing the likelihood of illness and promoting overall health, which translates to fewer sick days and a more robust work performance.
5. **Improved Physical Comfort**: Staying hydrated and choosing anti-inflammatory foods reduce bloating, fatigue, and stiffness, allowing you to work comfortably and stay focused on your tasks.

Prioritizing nutrition and hydration in the workplace is essential for maintaining peak performance, resilience, and well-being. By making mindful food and drink choices, you can sustain energy, improve focus, and enhance overall health. Simple steps, like choosing balanced meals, drinking water throughout the day, and including brain-boosting nutrients, can make a profound difference in your productivity and mood.

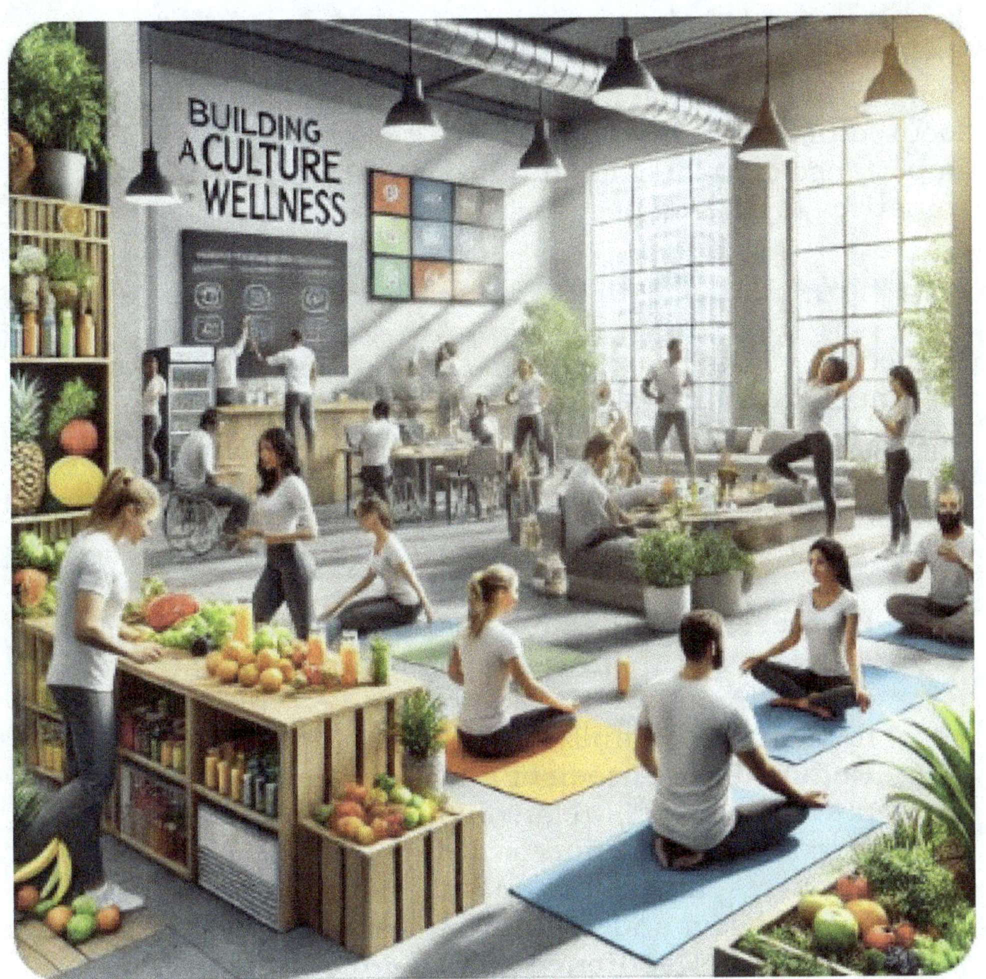

Chapter 6: Building a Culture of Wellness in the Workplace

A wellness-focused culture is integral to supporting employees' physical, mental, and emotional health in today's high-stress work environments. It's more than just perks and programs—it's about embedding well-being into the organization's values, policies, and daily practices. A strong culture of wellness creates a workplace where employees feel valued, empowered, and engaged, which ultimately contributes to organizational success.

In this expanded chapter, we'll explore deeper strategies for fostering a culture of wellness, from leadership and policy support to actionable programs and creating a wellness-focused physical environment. We'll also cover the importance of inclusivity and how to adapt wellness initiatives to diverse needs within the workforce.

Why a Culture of Wellness is Essential

In modern workplaces, chronic stress, sedentary behavior, and mental health challenges are common, impacting productivity, morale, and retention. A culture of wellness provides a foundation for addressing these issues by encouraging employees to adopt healthier lifestyles, manage stress effectively, and feel supported by their organization.

1. **Increased Engagement and Productivity**: Employees who feel that their well-being is prioritized are more engaged, motivated, and productive, which positively impacts the organization's bottom line.
2. **Reduced Absenteeism and Healthcare Costs**: By preventing stress-related illnesses, encouraging physical activity, and providing mental health resources, a wellness culture helps reduce absenteeism and healthcare costs.
3. **Enhanced Resilience and Reduced Burnout**: A wellness culture provides tools and resources that help employees manage stress and build resilience, reducing burnout and helping employees remain energized and engaged.
4. **Attraction and Retention of Top Talent**: A wellness culture aligns with the values of today's workforce, especially younger generations who prioritize work-life balance and mental health. This focus improves employee retention and enhances the organization's reputation.

To build a wellness culture that resonates with employees and creates lasting change, organizations need to focus on comprehensive wellness components that cover physical, mental, emotional, and environmental well-being.

1. Leadership Support and Advocacy

Wellness initiatives are most effective when they have the support of leaders who actively promote well-being as a company priority.

- **Role Modeling**: Leaders who prioritize their own well-being—taking breaks, managing stress, and participating in wellness activities—set a positive example, encouraging employees to do the same.
- **Allocating Resources and Budget**: Effective wellness programs require resources, including a dedicated budget, wellness staff, and access to services like mental health support and fitness programs. Leaders should demonstrate their commitment by ensuring these resources are available.
- **Communicating the Wellness Vision**: Leaders should communicate the organization's commitment to wellness by articulating a clear vision that aligns with the company's values and goals. This vision could include wellness priorities like mental health support, physical fitness, and work-life balance.

2. Comprehensive, Inclusive Wellness Programs

Wellness programs should cover multiple dimensions of health—physical, mental, and emotional—to address the diverse needs of employees. The most effective programs are inclusive and adaptable, making it easy for employees to participate.

- **Physical Wellness**: Offer fitness classes, walking clubs, or step challenges. Provide access to resources like gym memberships, on-site fitness centers, or wearable fitness devices. Creating incentives for movement, such as fitness challenges or rewards, also encourages participation.

- **Mental Health Support**: Make mental health a core component of wellness by providing access to counseling, therapy, and stress management workshops. Offering mental health days, promoting work-life balance, and destigmatizing mental health discussions contribute to a supportive environment.
- **Holistic Health Resources**: Wellness extends to nutrition, sleep, and stress management. Offer workshops or resources on topics like healthy eating, sleep hygiene, and time management. Providing access to wellness coaches or nutritionists can further support employees' overall health.

3. Policies that Support Work-Life Balance

Work-life balance is essential for long-term wellness, and policies that support it show employees that their personal lives and well-being are valued.

- **Flexible Work Arrangements**: Offer flexible hours, remote work options, or hybrid models. This flexibility allows employees to balance work with family and personal responsibilities, reducing stress and improving productivity.
- **Encouragement of Paid Time Off**: Encourage employees to use their vacation days, mental health days, and other paid time off. Leaders should set an example by taking time off themselves and respecting boundaries around work hours.
- **Limit Meeting Hours**: Schedule meetings only during certain hours (e.g., between 10 am and 3 pm) to allow employees uninterrupted time for focused work or personal needs. This policy respects employees' time and reduces meeting fatigue.

Encouraging movement throughout the day improves physical health, boosts energy levels, and promotes mental clarity. Movement can be as simple as taking breaks to stretch, walk, or stand.

- **Encourage Physical Activity Breaks**: Support movement by encouraging employees to take regular breaks for stretching, walking, or even a quick yoga session. Short activity breaks reduce muscle tension, improve circulation, and boost mental clarity.
- **Ergonomic Workstations and Standing Desks**: Invest in ergonomic furniture and provide standing desk options. These adjustments help prevent repetitive strain injuries and allow employees to change positions throughout the day.
- **Outdoor Activity Spaces**: Create outdoor spaces where employees can walk, exercise, or have walking meetings. Exposure to nature has been shown to reduce stress, improve mood, and enhance creativity.

5. Incorporate Mindfulness and Stress Management Programs

Mindfulness practices reduce stress, enhance focus, and improve resilience. By encouraging mindfulness, organizations help employees stay calm, focused, and balanced.

- **Mindfulness and Meditation Workshops**: Offer workshops on mindfulness, meditation, and breathing exercises. Guided sessions during work hours help employees manage stress, improve focus, and develop healthy coping skills.
- **Quiet Rooms or Wellness Spaces**: Designate spaces where employees can take a few minutes to meditate, reflect, or practice mindfulness. Quiet spaces provide a retreat from the demands of the workday and encourage intentional breaks.

- **Mindful Meeting Practices**: Start meetings with a brief moment of mindfulness, like a deep-breathing exercise or silent reflection, to set a focused, calm tone for discussion.

6. Foster Social Connections and a Sense of Community

Social support reduces stress and increases job satisfaction. A wellness culture fosters an environment where employees feel connected, valued, and part of a supportive team.

- **Team-Based Wellness Challenges**: Organize team-based wellness activities, like step challenges or healthy recipe contests, that encourage collaboration and friendly competition. Group activities promote social connections and make wellness fun.
- **Employee Resource Groups (ERGs)**: Support ERGs focused on wellness topics like mental health, nutrition, or fitness. ERGs provide peer support, build community, and create a safe space for discussing wellness issues.
- **Celebrate Wellness Achievements**: Recognize employees or teams who reach wellness milestones, such as completing a fitness challenge or achieving a personal wellness goal. Celebrating successes builds morale and reinforces the organization's commitment to wellness.

7. Provide Access to Wellness Education and Resources

Education empowers employees to make informed choices about their health. Providing diverse, accessible wellness resources demonstrates a commitment to lifelong health and learning.

- **Health Education Workshops**: Host regular workshops on relevant topics like nutrition, exercise, stress management, and sleep. These workshops equip employees with practical tips for improving their health.

- **Online Wellness Portal**: Provide access to a wellness portal with videos, articles, and resources that employees can access at any time. A wellness portal is especially useful for remote and hybrid employees.
- **Monthly Wellness Newsletters**: Distribute a wellness newsletter with tips on healthy living, updates on wellness programs, and highlights of wellness achievements within the company. A newsletter reinforces the company's commitment to wellness and keeps wellness top of mind.

8. Collect Feedback and Measure Success

Assessing wellness initiatives regularly helps organizations refine their programs, improve engagement, and demonstrate that employee input is valued.

- **Employee Feedback**: Use anonymous surveys, focus groups, or suggestion boxes to gather input on wellness programs, understand employees' needs, and identify areas for improvement.
- **Track Participation and Engagement Metrics**: Monitor participation rates in wellness programs, attendance at workshops, and engagement in wellness challenges. Tracking these metrics shows the impact of wellness programs on employee engagement and helps guide future initiatives.
- **Wellness Committees**: Form a wellness committee with representatives from different departments to ensure the program meets the diverse needs of employees. The committee can brainstorm new ideas, address challenges, and help implement initiatives.

Adapt Wellness Initiatives for Remote and Hybrid Workforces

As remote and hybrid work continues to evolve, organizations should adapt wellness programs to meet the needs of employees in various settings.

1. **Virtual Fitness and Mindfulness Sessions**: Offer virtual yoga, meditation, and fitness classes that remote employees can join from home. These sessions allow all employees to participate in wellness activities, regardless of location.
2. **Digital Wellness Challenges**: Create challenges that can be tracked digitally, like hydration goals, sleep improvements, or step counts. Online platforms make it easy to log progress and promote friendly competition.
3. **Provide Home Office Ergonomics Support**: Offer guidance on setting up an ergonomic home office or provide a stipend for ergonomic equipment. A comfortable workspace is essential for remote employees' physical wellness.
4. **Online Access to Wellness Resources**: Ensure remote employees have access to the same wellness resources as in-office employees, including counseling, mental health support, and wellness webinars. Offering online options ensures inclusivity in wellness initiatives.
5. **Foster Virtual Social Connections**: Host virtual coffee breaks, wellness check-ins, and team-building activities to maintain connections between remote and in-office employees. Building relationships remotely helps reduce isolation and builds community.

Long-Term Benefits of a Workplace Wellness Culture

A well-developed wellness culture has lasting effects that go beyond the individual to benefit the entire organization. Here are some of the long-term advantages of fostering wellness in the workplace:

1. **Higher Engagement and Morale**: Wellness-focused employees feel more valued and engaged, leading to improved morale, loyalty, and job satisfaction.
2. **Enhanced Productivity and Focus**: Healthier employees experience higher energy levels, better

focus, and increased resilience, which directly contribute to productivity.
3. **Reduced Healthcare Costs and Absenteeism**: Wellness programs prevent chronic health issues, reducing healthcare costs and minimizing absenteeism.
4. **Improved Organizational Resilience**: A wellness culture creates a resilient workforce that can navigate challenges and adapt to changes with greater ease.
5. **Stronger Employer Brand**: Organizations that prioritize wellness are more attractive to job seekers, building a reputation as a caring, forward-thinking employer that values work-life balance and mental health.

Building a culture of wellness in the workplace is a continuous, intentional process that requires leadership commitment, thoughtful policies, and a focus on employee needs. By implementing wellness programs, supporting work-life balance, fostering social connections, and creating an environment that prioritizes well-being, organizations can cultivate a happier, healthier, and more productive workforce. A wellness culture benefits everyone, leading to a positive, engaged workplace where employees feel valued and empowered to thrive.

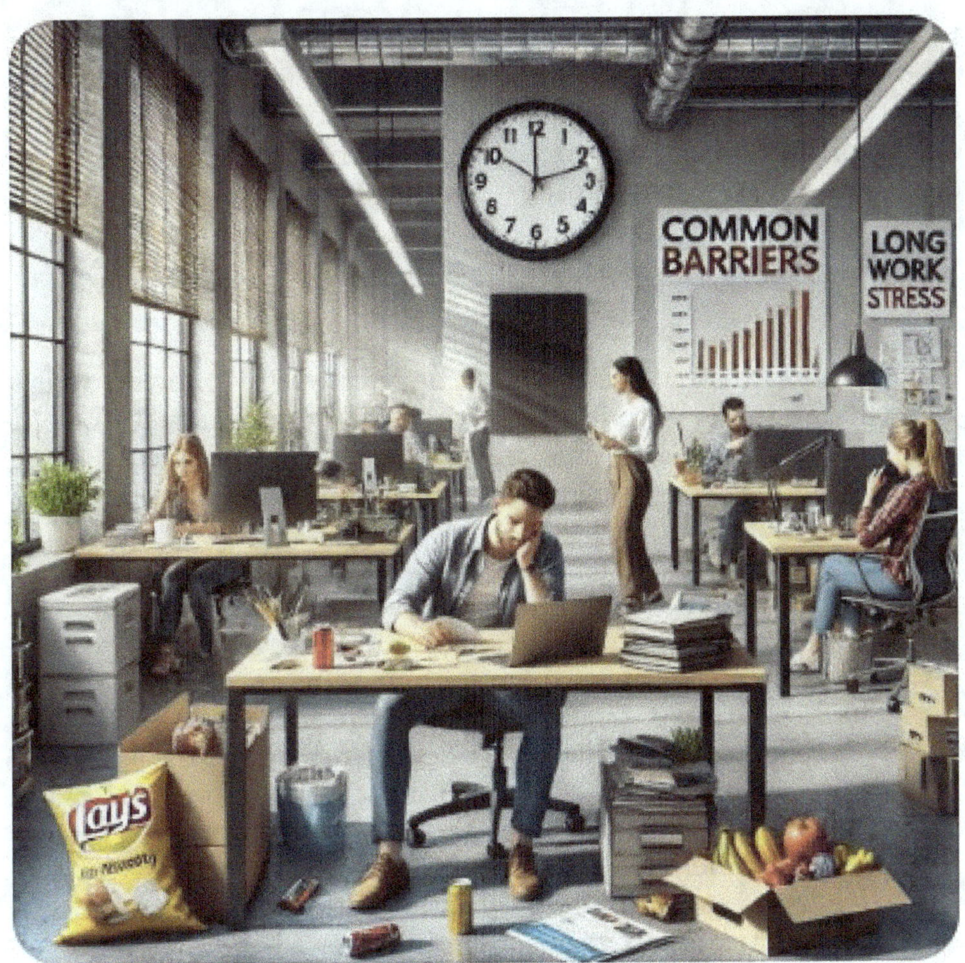

Chapter 7: Overcoming Common Barriers to Workplace Wellness

Building a culture of wellness in the workplace is a powerful investment, but it doesn't come without challenges. Common barriers, such as lack of time, limited resources, varying employee needs, and resistance to change, can hinder wellness initiatives and prevent employees from fully engaging. By identifying and proactively addressing these obstacles, organizations can create a more inclusive and accessible wellness culture that benefits everyone.

In this chapter, we'll explore some of the most common barriers to workplace wellness and provide actionable strategies to overcome them. From time management and resource limitations to overcoming skepticism and encouraging participation, we'll look at solutions to help organizations foster a supportive, health-focused environment where all employees can thrive.

1. **Time Constraints**: Many employees and managers feel that they simply don't have enough time to engage in wellness activities due to heavy workloads and tight schedules. For some, taking breaks for physical activity or mindfulness can feel like an interruption to productivity.
2. **Limited Resources and Budget**: Smaller organizations or departments may have limited budgets for wellness programs, making it challenging to offer perks like gym memberships, wellness workshops, or ergonomic equipment.
3. **Lack of Awareness or Understanding**: Some employees may not fully understand the benefits of wellness programs, leading to low engagement. Without clear communication, employees may view wellness initiatives as optional rather than valuable.
4. **Resistance to Change**: Employees who are used to traditional work routines may resist changes like incorporating movement breaks, flexible schedules, or mental health initiatives.
5. **Varying Employee Needs and Preferences**: A one-size-fits-all approach to wellness can fall short when employees have different health needs, fitness levels, schedules, or personal wellness goals. This can make it difficult to design programs that resonate with everyone.
6. **Physical Workspace Constraints**: Not all work environments are equipped to support wellness initiatives, especially if space is limited or employees are working remotely or in hybrid roles.

1. Time Constraints: Making Wellness Fit into Busy Schedules

Time is one of the most common barriers to wellness, but it's possible to integrate wellness into even the busiest schedules with a few strategic adjustments.

- **Encourage Micro-Breaks**: Promote the idea that wellness doesn't require long time commitments. Brief movement breaks, like a 5-minute stretch or a quick walk, can provide immediate benefits. Set reminders or encourage employees to schedule short breaks to move, breathe, or reset.
- **Incorporate Wellness into Daily Routines**: Help employees see wellness as part of their workday. Walking meetings, desk exercises, and mindfulness moments at the beginning of meetings can make wellness a seamless part of everyday routines.
- **Provide Flexible Wellness Options**: Offer flexible wellness programs that allow employees to participate when it suits their schedules. For instance, virtual yoga or meditation sessions that employees can join live or view on-demand provide flexibility for different time zones and work hours.
- **Lead by Example**: Leaders can set a powerful example by taking regular breaks for wellness activities and encouraging their teams to do the same. When employees see that management values well-being, they're more likely to prioritize it themselves.

2. Limited Resources and Budget: Creating Affordable Wellness Options

A wellness culture doesn't require a large budget. With creativity and resourcefulness, organizations can implement impactful wellness initiatives without overspending.

- **Leverage Free Resources**: Many online platforms offer free resources for fitness, mindfulness, and nutrition.

Consider sharing links to these resources, such as YouTube workout videos, guided meditation apps, or nutrition blogs, in company wellness newsletters or portals.

- **Encourage Walking Clubs or Group Walks**: Walking is a low-cost, effective way to improve physical and mental health. Organize walking groups for breaks, or encourage step challenges where employees can track their steps and compete for small prizes.
- **Utilize Internal Expertise**: Look for employees with wellness expertise who might be interested in leading a workshop, fitness class, or wellness talk. Internal resources can be valuable and help reduce program costs.
- **Partner with Local Businesses**: Collaborate with local fitness centers, wellness coaches, or health food stores to negotiate discounts or host workshops. Many businesses are open to partnerships and may offer special rates for group sessions or events.

3. Lack of Awareness or Understanding: Educating and Communicating the Value of Wellness

Employees may be less likely to engage in wellness activities if they don't fully understand the benefits or feel like the programs aren't for them. Clear, consistent communication can help bridge this gap.

- **Promote Wellness Education**: Host educational sessions on the benefits of wellness, covering topics like stress management, mental health, and the long-term impact of physical fitness. A greater understanding of wellness encourages participation and demonstrates the organization's commitment to employee health.
- **Highlight Success Stories**: Share testimonials from employees who have benefited from wellness programs. Success stories make wellness initiatives feel more relatable and can inspire others to get involved.

- **Make Information Easily Accessible**: Create a central wellness hub, whether it's a newsletter, intranet page, or app, where employees can access wellness information, resources, and program schedules. Accessible information increases awareness and engagement.
- **Provide Incentives for Participation**: Encourage initial participation by offering small incentives, like raffle entries, gift cards, or an extra day off for engaging in wellness activities. Incentives can attract attention and provide an entry point for hesitant employees.

4. Resistance to Change: Building Buy-In and Normalizing Wellness

Resistance to change can be a natural response to new initiatives. It's essential to build buy-in gradually and show how wellness programs fit into—and enhance—the workplace culture.

- **Start Small**: Introduce wellness programs gradually rather than overhauling routines all at once. Begin with simple changes, like encouraging hydration breaks or offering ergonomic adjustments, and expand based on employee feedback and comfort levels.
- **Engage Wellness Champions**: Identify wellness champions—employees who are passionate about health and wellness—who can advocate for programs, share their experiences, and motivate others. Peer support can make wellness initiatives more approachable.
- **Communicate the Value of Wellness to the Organization**: Emphasize how wellness programs align with company goals, such as increasing productivity, reducing absenteeism, and creating a positive work environment. When employees understand how wellness benefits the entire organization, they're more likely to support it.

- **Offer Training for Managers**: Provide managers with training on how to encourage wellness within their teams. Managers can play a key role in normalizing wellness practices by encouraging participation, supporting flexible schedules, and setting a healthy example.

5. Varying Employee Needs: Customizing Wellness for Inclusivity

A one-size-fits-all approach to wellness can miss the mark, as employees have different health goals, fitness levels, and preferences. Offering a range of options helps meet diverse needs.

- **Create a Variety of Program Options**: Offer a mix of physical, mental, and social wellness activities to cater to different interests. For example, some employees might prefer high-intensity fitness classes, while others might appreciate yoga or stress management workshops.
- **Encourage Self-Directed Wellness Goals**: Allow employees to set personal wellness goals and celebrate individual progress. This gives employees ownership of their wellness journey and helps them focus on what's most meaningful to them.
- **Provide Remote Wellness Options**: For hybrid and remote employees, offer virtual wellness activities, online classes, and resources that they can access from home. Ensuring remote workers have equal access to wellness resources makes programs more inclusive.
- **Gather Feedback Regularly**: Conduct regular surveys or focus groups to understand employee preferences and refine wellness programs. Gathering input allows the organization to adapt wellness offerings to better meet the changing needs of the workforce.

6. Physical Workspace Constraints: Making the Most of Limited Space

For companies with small or shared spaces, physical limitations can make it challenging to provide wellness facilities. However, there are creative ways to make space work for wellness.

- **Create Multi-Purpose Wellness Spaces**: If space is limited, create a flexible wellness area that can be used for different purposes, such as stretching, meditation, or quiet reflection. A small, dedicated area can have a big impact.
- **Encourage Outdoor Breaks**: If indoor space is limited, encourage employees to take breaks outdoors for fresh air and movement. Outdoor time can reduce stress, improve mood, and increase energy.
- **Implement Desk-Based Wellness**: For employees who work at desks, encourage desk-friendly exercises, stretches, and ergonomic adjustments that don't require additional space. Small tools, like resistance bands or stability cushions, can support wellness without taking up much room.
- **Support Remote Ergonomics**: For remote employees, provide guidelines for setting up an ergonomic workspace at home, or offer a stipend for ergonomic equipment. Ensuring remote workers have the resources they need supports their wellness regardless of location.

Encouraging Long-Term Engagement and Wellness Sustainability

Overcoming initial barriers is an essential step, but sustaining wellness initiatives and engagement requires ongoing attention and adaptation. Here are some strategies to encourage long-term engagement:

1. **Regularly Update Wellness Programs**: Periodically introduce new activities, workshops, or challenges to

keep wellness programs fresh and engaging. Variety can help maintain interest and appeal to different employees over time.

2. **Celebrate Small Wins and Milestones**: Recognize employees' wellness achievements, whether it's reaching a fitness goal, completing a wellness challenge, or consistently participating in mindfulness sessions. Celebrations, big or small, reinforce positive behavior and show appreciation for employee effort.

3. **Foster Peer Support Networks**: Create channels, like online wellness groups or peer mentoring, where employees can connect, share tips, and support each other. Social support encourages accountability and makes wellness a more enjoyable experience.

4. **Continue to Gather Feedback**: Regularly assess employee satisfaction with wellness programs through surveys or informal check-ins. Listening to feedback helps refine programs, making them more relevant and effective over time.

5. **Ensure Wellness is Accessible for All**: Make sure that wellness initiatives are accessible to all employees, regardless of role, location, or physical ability. This might involve offering both in-person and virtual options, adapting programs for accessibility, and ensuring flexibility.

Overcoming common barriers to workplace wellness requires creativity, flexibility, and an understanding of employees' unique needs. By addressing these obstacles head-on and making wellness accessible, organizations can foster an inclusive culture where wellness is seamlessly integrated into daily work life. When employees feel supported in their wellness journey, they're more likely to engage, stay motivated, and contribute positively to the workplace.

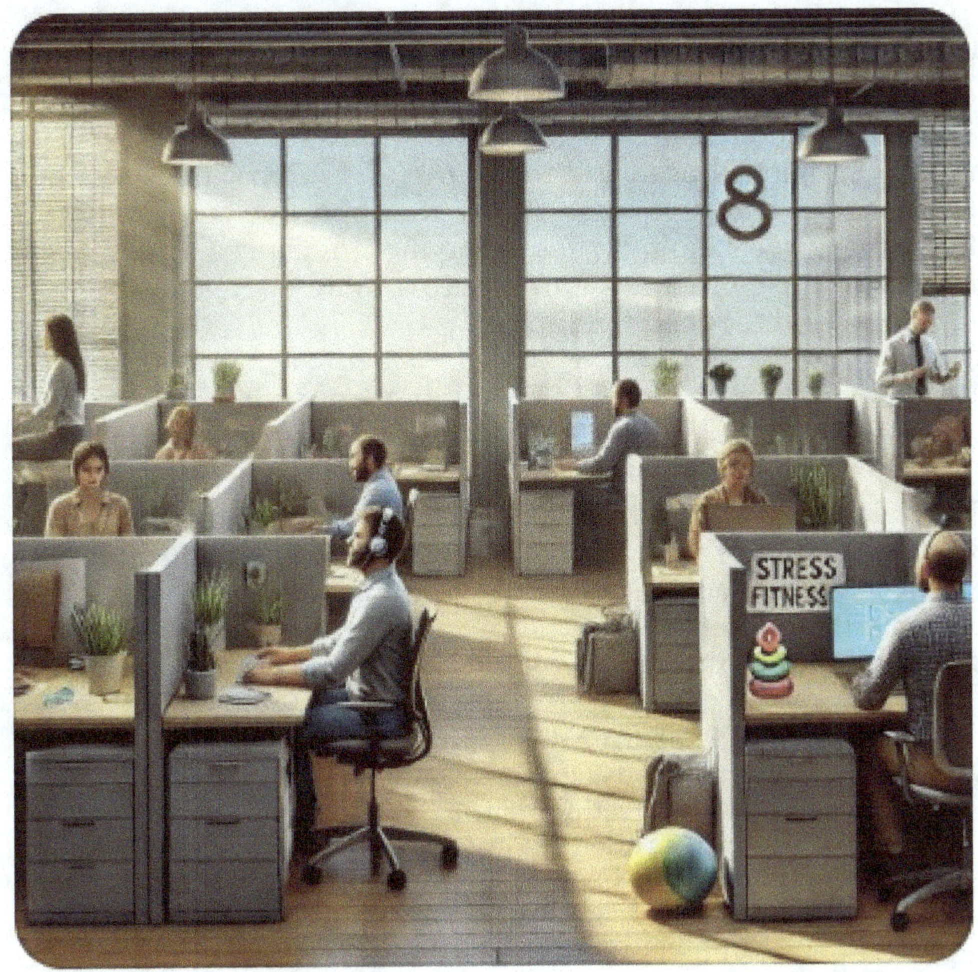

Chapter 8: Mental Fitness and Mindfulness in the Workplace

In today's fast-paced work environments, mental fitness and mindfulness are essential tools for building resilience, reducing stress, and improving focus. Mental fitness—defined as the ability to manage stress, maintain a positive mindset, and bounce back from challenges—is just as important as physical fitness for overall well-being and productivity. Mindfulness, which involves staying present and fully engaged in the moment, supports mental fitness by encouraging awareness, emotional regulation, and a greater sense of control.

This chapter explores the importance of mental fitness and mindfulness in the workplace, outlining the benefits for both employees and the organization. We'll examine strategies for integrating mental fitness and mindfulness into daily routines, discuss practical techniques, and provide insights into how organizations can create a supportive environment for mental well-being. By fostering mental fitness and mindfulness, companies can create a more engaged, resilient, and focused workforce.

The Importance of Mental Fitness and Mindfulness in the Workplace

Mental fitness and mindfulness have profound impacts on individual and organizational performance, contributing to reduced stress, enhanced focus, and improved decision-making. Here are some of the primary reasons why mental fitness and mindfulness are essential in the workplace:

1. **Stress Reduction and Emotional Regulation**:
   - Mental fitness enables employees to manage stress effectively, reducing the likelihood of burnout and improving their ability to handle challenges. Mindfulness supports emotional regulation by helping individuals remain calm and composed, even during high-stress situations.
2. **Enhanced Focus and Productivity**:
   - Mindfulness practices improve concentration, allowing employees to stay focused on tasks and make fewer mistakes. With improved mental clarity, employees can approach tasks more efficiently and creatively, enhancing overall productivity.
3. **Improved Resilience and Adaptability**:
   - Mental fitness fosters resilience, enabling employees to adapt to change, recover from setbacks, and approach challenges with a positive mindset. This resilience is essential in fast-paced environments where employees need to pivot quickly.
4. **Greater Job Satisfaction and Morale**:
   - When employees have the tools to manage stress and maintain a positive outlook, they experience higher job satisfaction and morale. This contributes to a

more positive workplace atmosphere and improved team dynamics.

5. **Enhanced Decision-Making and Problem-Solving**:
    o Mindfulness encourages a clear, balanced perspective, which improves decision-making and problem-solving. Employees who practice mindfulness are less reactive and more reflective, allowing them to approach complex problems with calm and focus.

Strategies for Building Mental Fitness and Mindfulness in the Workplace

To cultivate a mentally fit and mindful workplace, organizations should provide opportunities for employees to practice and develop these skills. Here are strategies for embedding mental fitness and mindfulness into the workday:

1. Encourage Mindfulness Practices During the Workday

Mindfulness practices don't have to be time-consuming; even brief moments of mindfulness can make a big difference. By incorporating mindfulness into daily routines, employees can reduce stress and improve their focus.

- **Mindful Breathing Exercises**: Encourage employees to take a few moments to practice mindful breathing. Techniques like "box breathing" (inhaling for a count of four, holding for four, exhaling for four, holding for four) can calm the mind and reduce anxiety. This can be especially helpful before meetings or presentations.
- **Mindfulness Moments Before Meetings**: Start meetings with a brief mindfulness exercise, such as a minute of silence or deep breathing. This practice helps employees center themselves, improve focus, and set a calm tone for the meeting.
- **Mindful Breaks**: Encourage employees to take short, mindful breaks throughout the day. This can include walking mindfully, stretching, or simply focusing on breathing for a few minutes. Mindful breaks are effective for resetting energy levels and reducing stress.

2. Incorporate Mental Fitness Training and Workshops

Mental fitness training helps employees build resilience, develop a positive mindset, and learn techniques to manage stress. Offering training programs and workshops on mental fitness can equip employees with tools for long-term mental well-being.

- **Resilience Training Workshops**: Host workshops that focus on resilience-building techniques, such as positive reframing, emotional regulation, and stress management. These skills empower employees to handle challenges more effectively and remain optimistic under pressure.
- **Mental Fitness Programs**: Provide programs that focus on core aspects of mental fitness, such as self-awareness, emotional intelligence, and cognitive flexibility. These programs teach employees how to adapt to changes, manage emotions, and maintain a positive mindset.
- **Mindfulness Training**: Offer introductory mindfulness sessions to teach employees about mindfulness principles and practices. These can include guided meditation, body scanning, and techniques for staying present. Regular mindfulness training reinforces healthy mental habits.

3. Create Dedicated Mindfulness Spaces

A dedicated space for mindfulness can serve as a retreat for employees to recharge and practice mindfulness during the workday. Even a small, quiet area can provide a place for meditation, reflection, or simply a few moments of calm.

- **Mindfulness Rooms or Quiet Areas**: Designate a quiet space in the office for mindfulness practices. Equip it with comfortable seating, calming decor, and resources like meditation cushions, blankets, or noise-canceling headphones. A peaceful environment encourages employees to take mindful breaks.

- **Outdoor Mindfulness Areas**: If space allows, create an outdoor mindfulness area where employees can meditate, do yoga, or simply enjoy a few moments in nature. Time spent outdoors has been shown to reduce stress and improve mental clarity, making it a valuable addition to mindfulness initiatives.
- **Virtual Mindfulness Spaces for Remote Employees**: For remote teams, provide access to virtual mindfulness spaces, such as guided meditation sessions or mindfulness apps. Offering remote options ensures that all employees can participate, regardless of location.

4. Encourage Journaling and Reflection

Journaling is an effective way to process emotions, gain self-awareness, and set goals. Encouraging employees to take time for personal reflection helps them develop mental clarity and reduce stress.

- **Reflection Time in the Workday**: Encourage employees to spend a few minutes each day journaling or reflecting. This could be at the start or end of the day, allowing employees to set intentions or reflect on achievements and challenges.
- **Gratitude Journals**: Introduce the practice of gratitude journaling, where employees write down things they are grateful for each day. Research shows that gratitude practices can improve mood, reduce stress, and increase job satisfaction.
- **Goal-Setting Journals**: Encourage employees to use journals for goal-setting, both personal and professional. Reflecting on progress and identifying next steps supports a positive mindset and fosters resilience.

5. Introduce Digital Tools for Mental Fitness and Mindfulness

Digital tools and apps make it easy for employees to engage in mental fitness and mindfulness activities at their convenience. By providing access to these resources, organizations can encourage regular practice.

- **Mindfulness Apps**: Apps like Headspace, Calm, and Insight Timer offer guided meditations, breathing exercises, and mindfulness practices that employees can use anytime. Consider offering access to these apps as part of the wellness program.
- **Mental Fitness Platforms**: Digital platforms like Lumosity and Happify offer games and activities designed to boost mental fitness by improving focus, memory, and stress management. Providing access to these platforms can make mental fitness more engaging and accessible.
- **Habit-Tracking Tools**: Encourage employees to use habit-tracking apps to build mental fitness and mindfulness routines. Apps like Habitica or Streaks help employees set and track goals, reinforcing consistency and progress in their mindfulness practices.

6. Encourage Regular Check-Ins and Self-Care Practices

Regular check-ins with oneself and supportive colleagues can reinforce mental fitness and mindfulness, promoting a positive, growth-oriented mindset.

- **Mindfulness Check-Ins**: Encourage employees to set reminders to check in with themselves throughout the day. Simple questions like, "How am I feeling?" or "What do I need right now?" help employees stay mindful of their emotional state and adjust accordingly.
- **Encourage Self-Care Practices**: Promote self-care practices like getting adequate sleep, taking time off when needed, and setting boundaries around work hours. Self-care reinforces mental resilience and prevents burnout, creating a balanced foundation for wellness.

- **Peer Support and Group Mindfulness Sessions**: Offer optional group mindfulness sessions or peer support groups where employees can connect and share their experiences with mindfulness. Group activities foster a sense of community and make mindfulness practices more approachable.

Benefits of Mental Fitness and Mindfulness for the Organization

Incorporating mental fitness and mindfulness into workplace wellness offers numerous benefits that positively impact organizational performance and culture:

1. **Reduced Stress and Burnout**:
   - Employees who practice mental fitness and mindfulness are better equipped to manage stress and reduce the risk of burnout. This leads to lower absenteeism, improved productivity, and a healthier workforce overall.
2. **Enhanced Creativity and Problem-Solving**:
   - Mindfulness encourages open-mindedness and the ability to see problems from new perspectives, enhancing creativity. When employees approach challenges with clarity and focus, they are more likely to generate innovative solutions.
3. **Improved Focus and Efficiency**:
   - By training the mind to stay present and focused, mindfulness reduces distractions and improves efficiency. Employees can accomplish more in less time, contributing to greater overall productivity.
4. **Increased Resilience and Adaptability**:
   - A mentally fit and mindful workforce is more resilient and adaptable to change. Employees who can manage stress and maintain a positive outlook are better equipped to handle transitions and challenges, fostering a resilient workplace culture.
5. **Stronger Team Relationships and Communication**:
   - Mindfulness practices encourage empathy, active listening, and open communication. This leads to stronger team relationships, improved collaboration, and a more supportive work environment.

Creating a culture that supports mental fitness and mindfulness requires commitment from leadership and integration into company values and practices. Here are ways to foster a mindfulness culture:

1. **Leadership Support and Participation**:
   - When leaders model mindfulness practices and mental fitness, they set a positive example for employees. Leaders who demonstrate these values encourage employees to prioritize mental well-being.
2. **Incorporate Mindfulness into Policies and Practices**:
   - Embed mindfulness into workplace policies, such as allowing flexible work hours, providing mental health days, and offering regular wellness check-ins. Policies that prioritize mental well-being make mindfulness an integral part of the work environment.
3. **Offer Continuous Learning Opportunities**:
   - Provide regular workshops, training sessions, and access to mindfulness resources to reinforce mental fitness skills. Continuous learning keeps employees engaged and motivated to build resilience and mindfulness over time.
4. **Celebrate Mindfulness Successes**:
   - Recognize and celebrate employees who actively participate in mindfulness practices or demonstrate resilience. Celebrating successes reinforces the importance of mental fitness and encourages a positive approach to well-being.

Mental fitness and mindfulness are essential components of a comprehensive wellness program, offering tools that empower employees to manage stress, improve focus, and build resilience. By incorporating these practices into daily routines, creating dedicated mindfulness spaces, and offering resources for continued learning, organizations can create a supportive environment that prioritizes mental well-being. A focus on mental fitness and mindfulness leads to reduced burnout, increased productivity, and a more positive workplace culture, fostering an engaged and resilient workforce ready to thrive in today's demanding work environments.

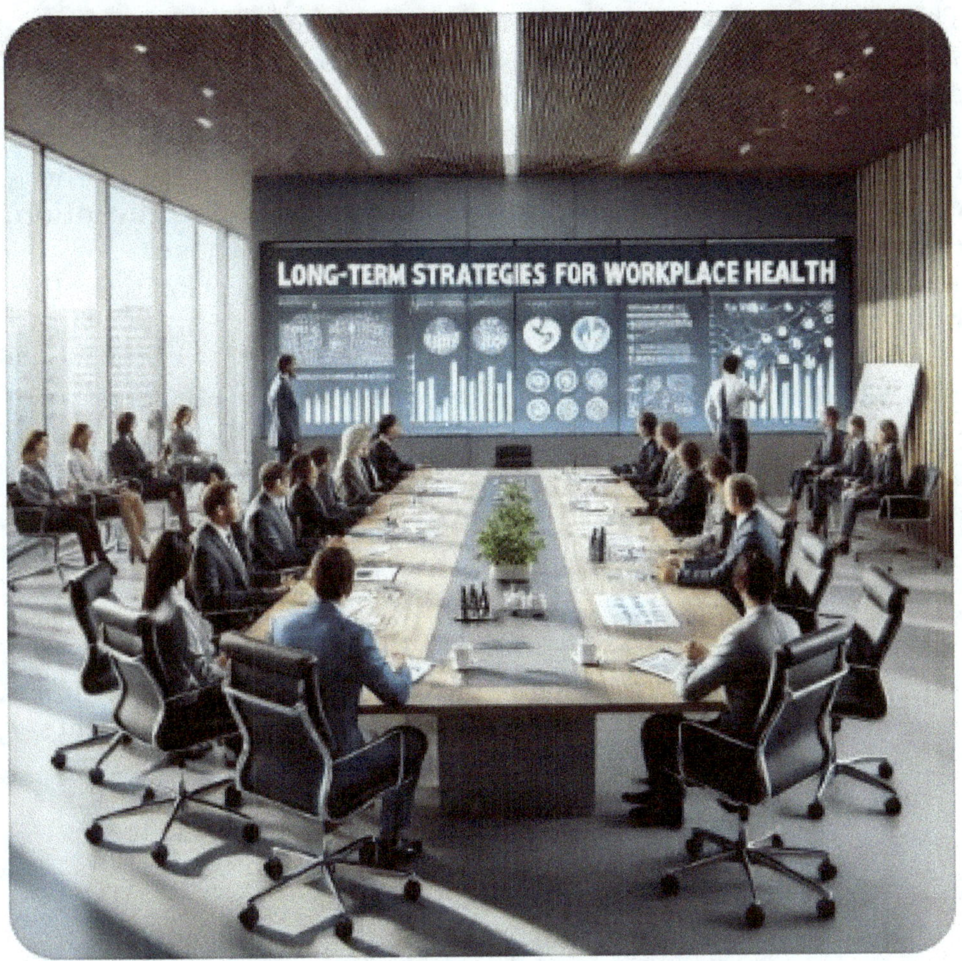

Chapter 9: Long-Term Strategies for Workplace Health

Building a healthy workplace isn't just about short-term wellness programs or one-time initiatives; it requires a long-term strategy that supports continuous well-being. Effective workplace health initiatives need to be sustainable, adaptable, and inclusive, evolving with the needs of the workforce and the organization. By implementing long-term strategies that prioritize physical, mental, and emotional well-being, companies can foster a resilient, healthy culture that supports employee engagement, reduces turnover, and enhances overall productivity.

This chapter provides a framework for developing long-term strategies that embed health and wellness into the fabric of an organization. We'll cover the principles of a sustainable wellness culture, outline practical approaches for maintaining engagement, and discuss ways to adapt to the changing needs of the workforce. With a focus on prevention, empowerment, and continuous improvement, these strategies aim to create a workplace that truly prioritizes the holistic health of its employees.

Why Long-Term Strategies are Essential for Workplace Health

1. **Sustainable Health Benefits**:
   - Long-term wellness strategies promote sustained improvements in health, reducing the risk of chronic conditions and improving quality of life for employees over time. Short-term programs often focus on immediate benefits, but long-term strategies address ongoing wellness and create lasting health benefits.
2. **Consistent Employee Engagement**:
   - When wellness becomes an integral part of the workplace culture, employees are more likely to engage consistently. A long-term approach shifts wellness from an optional perk to an essential component of the work environment, fostering greater buy-in and participation.
3. **Reduced Turnover and Improved Retention**:
   - Organizations that prioritize long-term health and wellness see higher retention rates. Employees are more likely to stay with a company that values their well-being and provides them with resources to lead a balanced, healthy lifestyle.
4. **Enhanced Organizational Performance**:
   - Healthy employees are more productive, focused, and resilient. Long-term wellness strategies contribute to improved job satisfaction, enhanced team dynamics, and greater overall organizational performance.

Building a lasting wellness culture requires a strategic focus on prevention, engagement, flexibility, and inclusivity. Below are the core elements of an effective long-term wellness strategy:

1. Prevention and Health Education

Prevention is at the heart of long-term wellness, reducing the likelihood of chronic conditions and promoting healthier lifestyles. By educating employees about prevention, organizations empower them to make informed health decisions.

- **Regular Health Screenings**: Offer regular health screenings to monitor key indicators like blood pressure, cholesterol, and blood glucose. Early detection of potential issues allows employees to take proactive steps and fosters a preventive health mindset.
- **Health Education Workshops**: Provide workshops on topics like nutrition, stress management, mental health, and sleep hygiene. Educational sessions equip employees with tools to make healthier choices and support their long-term well-being.
- **Disease Prevention Programs**: Implement targeted prevention programs that address lifestyle-related diseases such as diabetes, heart disease, and obesity. These programs can include resources on healthy eating, physical activity, and mental health support.
- **Ergonomics Education**: Educate employees on ergonomics and how to set up their workstations to prevent musculoskeletal issues. Provide regular training on posture, stretching exercises, and ergonomic equipment to prevent injuries.

2. Cultivating a Wellness-First Culture

A wellness-first culture places well-being at the core of the company's values, supporting long-term employee health through leadership support and integration into everyday work life.

- **Leadership Buy-In and Modeling**: When leaders prioritize wellness, they set a positive example for the entire organization. Leaders who participate in wellness activities, advocate for mental health, and take regular breaks create a culture where employees feel comfortable prioritizing their health.
- **Company Values and Policies**: Integrate wellness into the company's mission, values, and policies. For example, policies that support mental health days, flexible work hours, and boundaries around work hours reinforce the company's commitment to long-term well-being.
- **Regular Wellness Communication**: Keep wellness top of mind with regular communication, such as newsletters, wellness tips, or updates on health initiatives. Ongoing communication helps reinforce the importance of wellness and keeps employees engaged.
- **Recognition of Wellness Achievements**: Recognize employees who actively participate in wellness initiatives or reach personal health milestones. Celebrating achievements shows that the organization values health and well-being and encourages ongoing participation.

3. Flexible Wellness Programs and Adaptability

Long-term wellness programs must be flexible and adaptable to meet the diverse needs of employees as they change over time. Flexibility in wellness programs ensures inclusivity and supports employees at different stages of their wellness journey.

- **Diverse Wellness Offerings**: Offer a wide range of wellness options, including fitness classes, mindfulness sessions, nutrition counseling, and health coaching. Diverse options cater to different interests and make wellness more accessible to all employees.
- **Hybrid and Remote Wellness Options**: As remote work becomes more common, it's important to offer virtual wellness programs that employees can access from anywhere. Provide online resources, virtual fitness classes, and remote-friendly wellness activities to ensure inclusivity.
- **Personalized Wellness Plans**: Encourage employees to set individual wellness goals and provide resources to support them. Personalized wellness plans allow employees to focus on their unique health priorities and create a more meaningful wellness experience.
- **Adaptable Program Feedback and Updates**: Regularly gather feedback from employees to understand which programs are effective and make necessary adjustments. A responsive approach to feedback keeps wellness initiatives relevant and aligned with employee needs.

4. Empowering Employees Through Self-Care and Autonomy

Long-term wellness strategies should empower employees to take control of their health. Encouraging self-care and providing employees with the autonomy to make wellness decisions fosters a proactive approach to well-being.

- **Self-Care Days and Mental Health Support**: Offer self-care days or mental health days, allowing employees to take time for themselves without needing a specific reason. Self-care days empower employees to prioritize their mental health, reducing burnout and improving long-term well-being.
- **Encourage Work-Life Balance**: Implement policies that support work-life balance, such as flexible work hours, boundaries around after-hours communication, and remote work options. A focus on work-life balance

helps employees manage stress and maintain overall health.

- **Promote Autonomy in Wellness Choices**: Empower employees to choose their wellness activities based on their preferences and needs. Offering options, rather than mandating specific programs, increases engagement and makes wellness more enjoyable.
- **Encourage Goal Setting and Accountability**: Support employees in setting wellness goals, whether related to physical fitness, mental health, or personal growth. Providing resources like wellness coaches or goal-setting workshops helps employees stay accountable and motivated.

5. Creating an Inclusive Wellness Environment

An inclusive wellness environment accommodates the diverse needs, backgrounds, and abilities of all employees. Long-term wellness strategies should embrace inclusivity to ensure everyone feels supported in their wellness journey.

- **Accessible Wellness Options**: Provide wellness options that accommodate employees of all fitness levels, abilities, and ages. This can include adaptive fitness classes, mental health resources, and tailored programs for different demographics.
- **Culturally Sensitive Wellness Programs**: Offer wellness programs that respect and celebrate cultural diversity. This might include offering a range of wellness resources that consider dietary preferences, religious practices, and cultural norms.
- **Inclusive Wellness Spaces**: Create physical and virtual wellness spaces that are accessible to all employees. Ensure that wellness rooms are comfortable, accessible, and equipped with resources for both physical and mental wellness.
- **Diverse Health and Wellness Content**: Include diverse perspectives in wellness materials and resources. Representing a variety of backgrounds and experiences promotes inclusivity and ensures that all

employees feel seen and valued in the wellness program.

Evaluating and Sustaining Long-Term Wellness Programs

Long-term wellness success depends on continuous evaluation and adaptation. Regularly assessing the impact of wellness programs ensures that they remain effective and continue to meet the evolving needs of the workforce.

1. **Use Data to Track Health Trends and Outcomes**:
   - Collect data on health outcomes, program participation, and employee satisfaction to monitor wellness trends. Reviewing this data helps the organization identify areas of improvement and adapt programs to maintain engagement.
2. **Gather Employee Feedback Regularly**:
   - Conduct surveys, focus groups, or feedback sessions to understand employee experiences and preferences. Regular feedback ensures that wellness initiatives align with the needs and desires of employees.
3. **Benchmark Against Industry Standards**:
   - Benchmark wellness programs against industry standards and best practices. Comparing programs with other organizations helps identify gaps, set realistic goals, and ensure that wellness initiatives are competitive and effective.
4. **Create a Cycle of Continuous Improvement**:
   - Use evaluation data to create a continuous improvement plan. Regularly update wellness programs, introduce new activities, and refine offerings to keep the program dynamic and relevant.
5. **Celebrate and Communicate Successes**:
   - Regularly share the successes of wellness programs with employees, including data on improved health outcomes, reduced absenteeism, or employee testimonials. Celebrating successes reinforces the value of wellness and encourages continued participation.

Implementing long-term wellness strategies yields numerous benefits for both employees and the organization:

1. **Improved Health and Reduced Healthcare Costs**:
   - A consistent focus on prevention and wellness leads to healthier employees and fewer chronic health issues. This results in lower healthcare costs for both employees and the organization.
2. **Higher Employee Engagement and Retention**:
   - Organizations with a strong wellness culture see higher employee engagement and retention. When employees feel supported in their well-being, they are more loyal, motivated, and committed to the organization.
3. **Enhanced Organizational Resilience**:
   - A wellness-focused organization fosters resilience, helping employees cope with challenges, adapt to change, and recover from setbacks. This adaptability creates a stronger, more resilient workforce.
4. **Greater Productivity and Focus**:
   - Healthy employees are more focused, energized, and productive. Long-term wellness programs contribute to improved job performance, fewer mistakes, and enhanced creativity.
5. **Positive Employer Brand and Attraction of Talent**:
   - A long-term wellness strategy enhances the organization's reputation as an employer that values health and well-being. This positive brand image attracts top talent, especially those who prioritize work-life balance and well-being.

Building a long-term strategy for workplace health requires a commitment to prevention, flexibility, inclusivity, and continuous improvement. By embedding wellness into the culture and providing employees with the tools and resources to prioritize their well-being, organizations can create a sustainable, supportive environment where employees thrive. Long-term wellness programs aren't just beneficial for individual health—they're essential for building a resilient, engaged, and productive workforce.

Conclusion: Building a Culture of Health and Well-Being in the Workplace

Creating a workplace that prioritizes wellness is no longer a nice-to-have; it's an essential strategy for fostering a resilient, engaged, and productive workforce. By embedding wellness into the organization's culture, offering a variety of wellness initiatives, and continuously evolving with employee needs, companies can support their employees' physical, mental, and emotional well-being. This book has outlined the foundations of an effective wellness program—from creating flexible, inclusive wellness options to incorporating physical activity, mental health support, mindfulness practices, and ergonomics into daily routines.

A successful wellness culture requires a holistic approach, where wellness isn't seen as a one-time initiative but as a core component of organizational values and day-to-day operations. A culture of health doesn't come overnight; it takes thoughtful planning, regular engagement, and a commitment to continuous improvement. By leveraging data, feedback, and insights into employee needs, organizations can refine their wellness programs, adapt to changing circumstances, and make wellness accessible to all.

The benefits of prioritizing workplace wellness go beyond healthier employees. A robust wellness culture contributes to reduced healthcare costs, lower turnover, higher engagement, and improved overall performance. Employees who feel supported in their well-being are more motivated, creative, and loyal to their employers, creating a workplace that attracts and retains top talent.

As the nature of work continues to evolve, so too should our approach to employee wellness. The strategies and insights in this book are a starting point for building a healthier, more balanced, and more supportive workplace. By committing to wellness as a journey rather than a destination, organizations can cultivate a thriving environment where both employees and the business can grow and succeed together.

Remember, a healthy workplace is not just about better work outcomes—it's about creating a space where people feel valued, empowered, and inspired. By fostering wellness in the workplace, you are not only investing in the future of your organization but in the well-being of each individual within it.

Appendix: Resources for Workplace Wellness

This appendix provides a curated list of resources to support workplace wellness, covering areas such as mental health, physical fitness, ergonomics, and general well-being. These resources include online tools, apps, organizations, and guides to help you build, maintain, and evolve a culture of wellness within your organization.

Mental Health and Mindfulness

1. **Mindfulness Apps**:
   - *Headspace* – Offers guided meditations, mindfulness exercises, and sleep aids tailored to reduce stress and increase focus.
   - *Calm* – Provides guided meditation, sleep stories, breathing exercises, and music to support relaxation.
   - *Insight Timer* – A free app with thousands of meditations and guided practices, including live sessions with mindfulness experts.
2. **Mental Health Organizations**:
   - *National Alliance on Mental Illness (NAMI)* – Provides educational resources, support groups, and tools for promoting mental health in the workplace.
   - *Mental Health America (MHA)* – Offers resources, screenings, and toolkits for promoting mental health awareness and support.
3. **Mindfulness Training**:
   - *Search Inside Yourself Leadership Institute (SIYLI)* – Offers mindfulness and emotional intelligence training for workplaces, based on a program developed at Google.
   - *Mindful Schools* – Provides online courses and training programs for incorporating mindfulness practices into the workplace.

Physical Fitness and Activity

1. **Fitness and Wellness Apps**:
   - *MyFitnessPal* – Tracks nutrition, exercise, and hydration, making it easy for employees to set and reach health goals.

- o *Nike Training Club* – Offers free workouts across a variety of fitness levels, including strength, yoga, and high-intensity interval training.
  - o *Strava* – A tracking app for walking, running, and biking challenges, allowing employees to connect and share their progress.
2. **Wearable Technology**:
  - o *Fitbit* – Tracks steps, heart rate, and physical activity, ideal for step challenges and fitness tracking in wellness programs.
  - o *Garmin* – Offers wearable devices for tracking a range of health metrics, including sleep, stress levels, and heart rate variability.
3. **Group Fitness Resources**:
  - o *ClassPass* – A subscription service that provides access to thousands of gyms and fitness studios, offering flexibility and variety.
  - o *Peloton Digital Membership* – Provides on-demand fitness classes, including cycling, running, strength, and yoga, that can be accessed anywhere.

Ergonomics and Workspace Setup

1. **Ergonomic Guidelines and Resources**:
  - o *Occupational Safety and Health Administration (OSHA)* – Offers ergonomic guidelines for office settings and other work environments, with resources for creating safe, comfortable workspaces.
  - o *Cornell University Ergonomics Web* – Provides ergonomic tips, assessment tools, and best practices for office setup and posture.
2. **Ergonomic Tools and Equipment**:
  - o *Uplift Desk* – Provides standing desks, adjustable desks, and ergonomic office furniture to promote healthy posture and movement.
  - o *Ergotron* – Offers a range of ergonomic products, including sit-stand workstations, monitor mounts, and active seating options.
3. **Online Ergonomic Assessments**:
  - o *ErgoApp* – An online assessment tool that helps identify ergonomic risks and provides personalized recommendations for workstation adjustments.

- o *WorkRite Ergonomics* – Offers virtual ergonomic assessments and guidance on setting up an ergonomic home or office workspace.

1. **Employee Assistance Programs (EAPs)**:
    - o *ComPsych* – Provides a comprehensive EAP that includes counseling, financial wellness, legal assistance, and work-life support.
    - o *LifeWorks* – Offers an integrated EAP with resources for mental health, financial wellness, and family support, along with a wellness app.
2. **Wellness Program Platforms**:
    - o *Virgin Pulse* – A wellness platform that offers custom wellness programs, fitness challenges, and incentives to encourage participation.
    - o *Wellable* – A customizable wellness platform that includes a variety of health and wellness challenges, tracking options, and rewards.
3. **General Health and Wellness Resources**:
    - o *Centers for Disease Control and Prevention (CDC) Workplace Health Promotion* – Provides resources, toolkits, and guides for developing a workplace wellness program focused on prevention and health education.
    - o *The World Health Organization (WHO) Workplace Health Toolkit* – Offers resources and guides for creating a healthy, safe workplace, with a focus on physical and mental well-being.

Team-Building and Wellness Challenges

1. **Virtual Wellness Challenges**:
    - o *MoveSpring* – A platform for team-based challenges like step counting, activity tracking, and custom fitness challenges, ideal for virtual and hybrid workplaces.
    - o *ChallengeRunner* – A challenge platform that tracks wellness activities and encourages friendly competition among employees.

2. **Team Building and Engagement Tools**:
   - *Kahoot!* – A game-based learning platform that can be used for wellness quizzes, team challenges, and fun learning activities related to health.
   - *Slack or Microsoft Teams* – Integrate wellness-focused channels or bots that provide daily wellness tips, reminders for breaks, and space for team motivation.
3. **Step-Tracking Tools and Apps**:
   - *Pacer* – A step-tracking app that enables groups to create and participate in step challenges, promoting regular movement.
   - *MapMyWalk* – A fitness app that allows employees to track their walking routes, set goals, and share progress with colleagues.

Learning and Development in Wellness

1. **Professional Certifications in Wellness**:
   - *National Wellness Institute (NWI)* – Offers certifications such as Certified Wellness Practitioner (CWP) for individuals seeking professional training in workplace wellness.
   - *American College of Sports Medicine (ACSM)* – Provides certifications for wellness coaches and health promotion specialists, focusing on corporate wellness skills.
2. **Online Courses and Wellness Workshops**:
   - *Coursera* – Offers online courses on wellness topics such as mindfulness, nutrition, exercise science, and stress management from leading universities.
   - *edX* – Provides wellness-related courses, including topics on mental health, workplace ergonomics, and public health, that employees can access for personal growth.
3. **Wellness Webinars and Virtual Events**:
   - *Wellness Council of America (WELCOA)* – Offers webinars, workshops, and online events focused on workplace wellness trends and best practices.
   - *Employee Wellness Solutions Network (EWSN)* – Provides webinars, workshops, and custom wellness programs for corporate clients, focusing on mental and physical health.

1. **Wellness Benchmarking and Trends**:
   - *Global Wellness Institute (GWI)* – Provides insights into global wellness trends, data, and resources on the latest developments in workplace wellness.
   - *Gallup's Workplace Wellness Insights* – Regularly publishes studies on employee engagement, well-being, and the impact of wellness programs on organizational performance.
2. **Research on Workplace Wellness and ROI**:
   - *Harvard T.H. Chan School of Public Health – Workplace Health Research* – Publishes research on the benefits and ROI of workplace wellness programs, with resources for organizations to measure success.
   - *RAND Workplace Wellness Programs Study* – Offers insights into the effectiveness of wellness programs, including data on health outcomes, cost savings, and employee engagement.
3. **Policy and Legal Resources for Workplace Wellness**:
   - *Society for Human Resource Management (SHRM) – Wellness Policies* – Provides policy templates, legal guidelines, and best practices for implementing wellness programs within organizational policies.
   - *Employee Benefits Security Administration (EBSA)* – A branch of the U.S. Department of Labor, offering guidelines and compliance information for companies offering wellness benefits as part of their health plans.